Hand
Reflexology

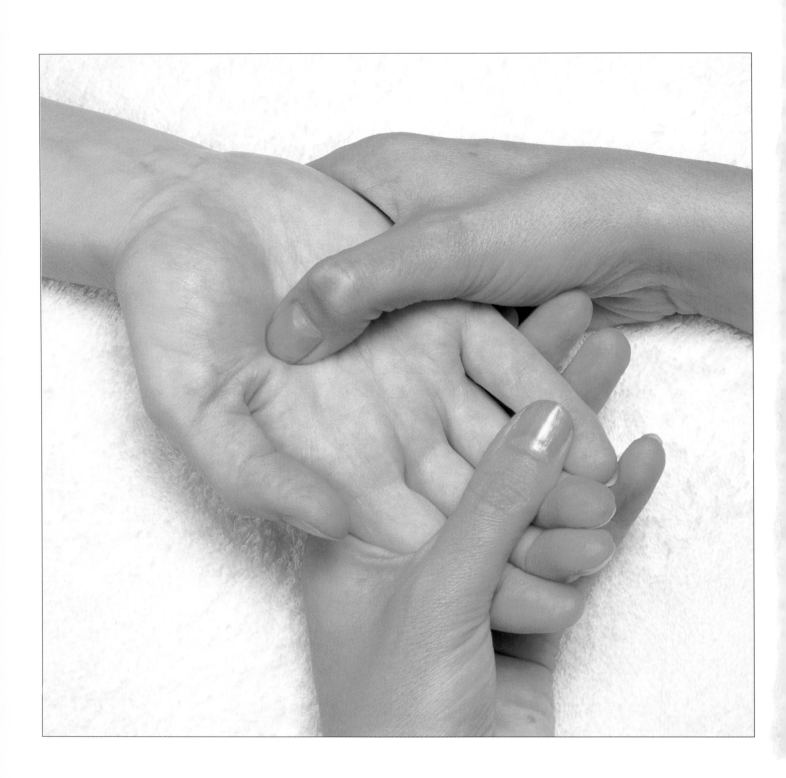

Hand Reflexology

A practical introduction

DENISE WHICHELLO BROWN

Eagle
Editions

A QUANTUM BOOK

Published by Eagle Editions Ltd
11 Heathfield
Royston
Hertfordshire SG8 5BW

ISBN 1-86160-391-6

QUMAIHA

This book is produced by
Quantum Publishing
6 Blundell Street
London N7 9BH

Printed in Singapore by
Star Standard Industries Pte Ltd

contents

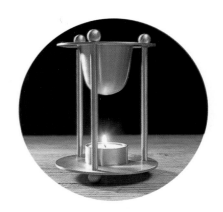

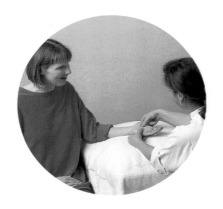

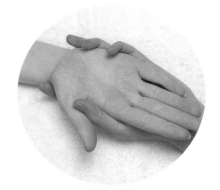

introduction to
Hand Reflexology

Although many books have been written about reflexology, most of them concentrate on reflexology of the feet, rather than the hand. This book serves as an introduction to the art of hand reflexology, and contains easy-to-follow instructions on the basic techniques, as well as providing step-by-step sequences for each hand and details on treating a variety of common ailments. There is also a very comprehensive section on self-treatment.

Unlike the more widely practised foot reflexology, the beauty of hand reflexology is that it can be carried out absolutely anywhere. Standing up, waiting for a bus or train, sitting down whilst travelling to work, in your lunch or tea break or when relaxing in the evening. What's more it is extremely good for you. Hand reflexology helps you to relax, boosts the immune system, improves the circulation, aids the elimination of toxins, improves mental function, boosts energy levels and much more besides.

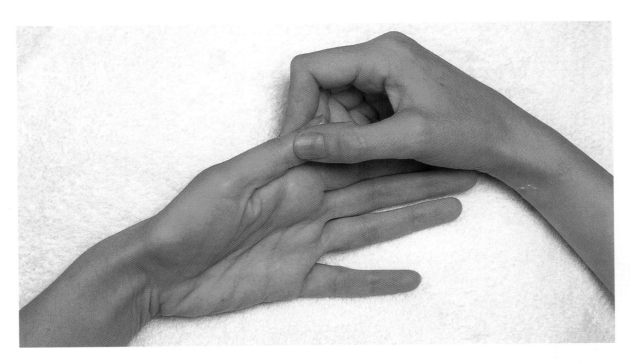

Hand reflexology is ideally suited to self-treatment.

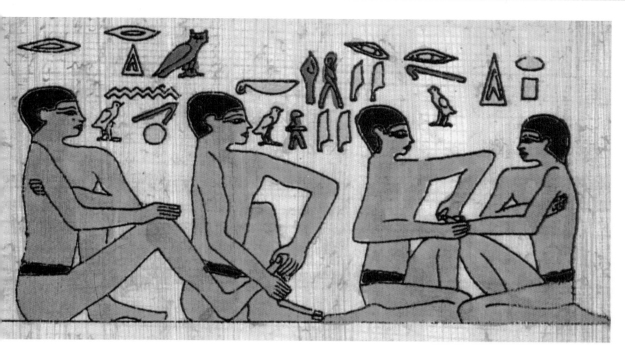

*Illustration from the tomb of Ankmahor in Saqqara, Egypt.
Dated around 2330 BC.*

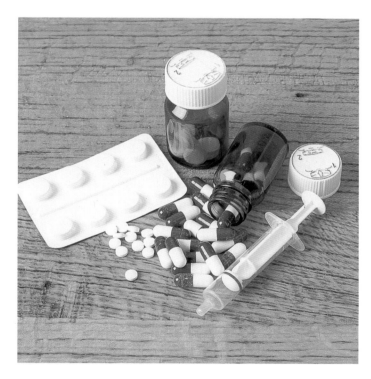

*Reflexology has found widespread acceptance as a complement
to conventional medicines.*

A Brief History of Reflexology

Reflexology is an ancient therapeutic treatment in evidence
thousands of years ago. A painting discovered in Saqqara, Egypt,
in the tomb of Ankmahor, the physician shows a reflexology
treatment in progress. This painting dates back to about 2330
BC. There is also evidence that reflexology was commonly
practised in China.

Reflexology as we know it today originated with the work of
the American physician Doctor William Fitzgerald (1872-1942)
who developed his 'zone therapy' and divided the body into ten
longitudinal zones.

Doctor Joseph Shelby-Riley and his wife, true believers in
Doctor Fitzgerald's work, wrote several books including 'Zone
Therapy Simplified' (1919). Doctor Riley is particularly
renowned as the teacher of Eunice Ingham, who is regarded by
many to be the founder and mother of modern reflexology. In
1938 she published 'Stories the Feet Can Tell' followed by the
sequel 'Stories the Feet Have Told'–two classic texts which are
still used by reflexologists today. Eunice Ingham died in 1974 at
the age of 85, and it is true to say that it is due to her efforts that
reflexology is so popular today. It is a fast-growing therapy
worldwide and it has become increasingly accepted over the years
by practitioners of conventional medicines. There are doctors,
nurses, osteopaths, chiropractors, acupuncturists and
homoeopaths practising today who have incorporated the art of
reflexology into their treatments.

Hand Reflexology?

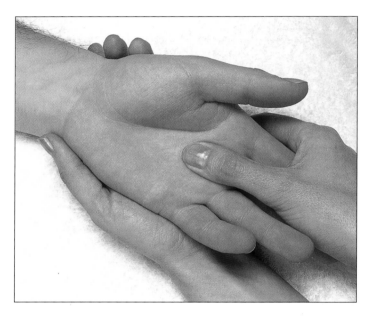

Reflex points in the hand mirror specific organs and structures of the body.

Hand reflexology is a method of applying pressure through the fingers and thumbs on the reflex areas of the hands. These reflex areas are found on all parts of the hands and they correspond to the organs, glands and structures of the body. The hands can be seen as a mirror of the body — the right hand reflects the right hand side of the body while the left hand reflects the left hand side.

Reflexology is a simple, non-invasive natural therapy, which stimulates the inner healing forces within the body, bringing about physical, mental and emotional well-being. Whether you have a specific health problem or are just looking for a way to relieve tension and promote optimum health, reflexology is of excellent therapeutic value.

Hand reflexology is completely safe provided that it is administered correctly. As long as a particular reflex is not overworked there is no danger of over-stimulation which can cause excessive elimination and unpleasant side-effects. It can be used on everyone from young babies to the elderly.

IMPORTANT:

- Reflexology should NEVER be used to diagnose medical conditions. A medical diagnosis should only be carried out by a qualified doctor.

- When giving a reflexology treatment, you must NEVER promise to 'cure' an ailment, nor should you use reflexology to give false hope. However, everyone WILL benefit from reflexology.

- Reflexology should NOT be used instead of orthodox medicine. The advice of a medically qualified doctor should always be sought. However, reflexology and orthodox medicine work well when used together.

- Reflexology should NOT be classed as a medical treatment.

- Reflexology is NOT like an acupuncture treatment. Acupuncturists talk about meridians whereas reflexologists use zones. Acupuncture is an extremely complex subject, which can take four years of full-time study. It can be very dangerous if not practised properly.

The Bony Structure of the Hands

There are 27 bones making up each hand and wrist. These are:

8 CARPALS (wrist bones) arranged in two rows. They are known as the trapezium (four-sided), trapezoid (four-sided), capitate, hamate (hook shaped), scaphoid (like a boat), lunate (resembles a crescent moon), triquetral, pisiform (pea-shaped).

5 METACARPALS, which form the palm of the hand. The heads of these bones make the knuckles.

14 PHALANGES, which are the finger and thumb bones. The thumb has two phalanges whereas the fingers have three.

The bones of the hand and wrist are held in place by an enormous number of muscles, tendons and ligaments. There is a rich supply of nerve endings in the hands, which make them very sensitive.

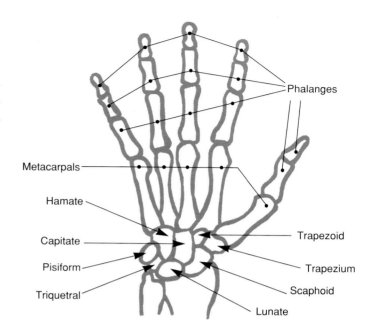

PRINCIPLES OF REFLEXOLOGY

The Ten Longitudinal Zones

Ten Longitudinal Zones

According to reflexology the body can be divided into ten longitudinal zones which run the length of body from the tips of the toes to the head and out to the fingertips and vice versa. If an imaginary line is drawn through the centre of the body there are five zones to the right of this mid-line and five zones to the left.

Zone one runs from the big toe, up the leg and centre of the body to the head and then down to the thumb.

Zone two runs from the second toe up to the head and then down to the index finger.

Zone three extends from the third toe up to the head, then down to the third finger and so on.

All organs and parts of the body, which lie within the same zone are related to each other. If any part of a zone is stimulated in the hand this will affect the entire zone throughout the body.

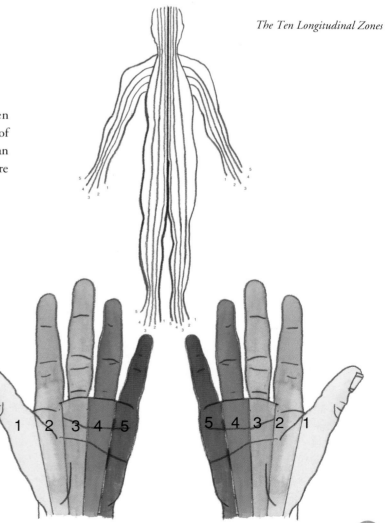

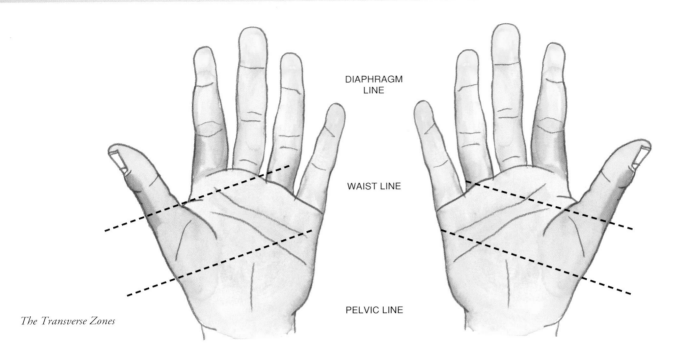

DIAPHRAGM
LINE

WAIST LINE

PELVIC LINE

The Transverse Zones

Transverse Zones

Reflexology also divides the hands (and feet) into transverse or horizontal sections.

1) The first transverse zone – the diaphragm line – on the hand is located just below the padded area beneath the fingers. All the organs above the diaphragm on the body are found here.

2) The second transverse zone – waist line – runs from the base of the web between the thumb and index finger where the thumb joins the hand across the hand.

3) The third transverse zone – pelvic line – circles the wrist.

The transverse zones and the longitudinal zones help us to describe the position of the reflexes on the hands.

Why Hand Reflexology?

Foot reflexology is the most popular form of reflexology and if you made an appointment to see a professional reflexologist the treatment would take place primarily on the feet. Hand reflexology is usually recommended as a self-help treatment to reinforce the work of the reflexologist.

However, times are changing and there is an increasing interest in the use of hand reflexology as the primary treatment. It has often been found that hand reflexology is a highly effective treatment, and sometimes patients have responded more quickly to hand reflexology than to foot reflexology. The best practices today generally use a combination of hand and foot reflexology and the results are excellent.

There are some occasions when it is impossible to administer foot reflexology and then working the hands becomes a necessity. Such circumstances include:

1) If the foot is injured — e.g. fractures; sprains etc.
2) If the foot is infected.
3) If the foot has been amputated.
4) If a person is too shy or embarrassed to expose his/her feet.
5) If the feet are extremely sensitive and cannot be touched without causing discomfort.
6) If the foot or part of the foot is very inflamed — e.g. gout in the big toe.
7) If foot reflexology has not previously worked, or progress is very slow.
8) If self-treatment is required.

Getting started

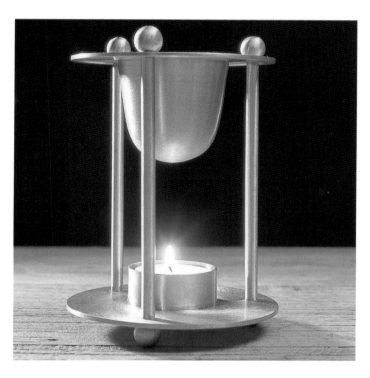

An oil burner can help provide soft lighting, as well as a calming aroma.

CREATING A SUITABLE ATMOSPHERE

Although the beauty of giving a hand reflexology treatment is that it can be carried out anywhere, if you create the right ambience you will achieve optimum results.

Ideally the surroundings should be as peaceful and calm as possible. Telephones ringing and children banging on the door to attract your attention ARE not conducive to relaxation, so remove as many distractions as possible, and ensure that you will not be disturbed. Some people enjoy silence during their treatment whilst others will prefer to listen to some soft relaxation music. It is up to the individual.

The room should be warm and inviting with soft and subdued lighting. Essential oils can be burned prior to the treatment. Particularly relaxing oils include lavender, chamomile, frankincense, sandalwood and ylang ylang. A vase of fresh flowers or some softly scented pot pourri will also enhance the environment.

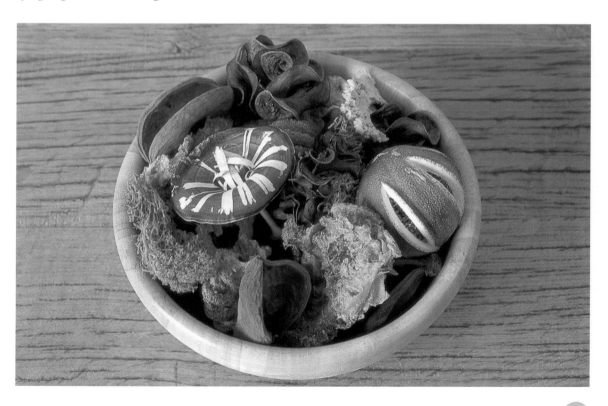

The gentle scent of pot pourri can enhance the atmosphere.

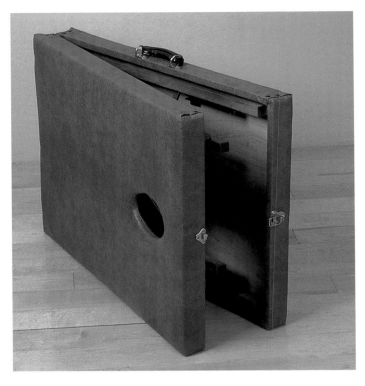

A massage couch is a useful purchase for frequent treatments, but not essential.

POSITIONS FOR WORKING

Correct positioning of the receiver is an important factor in the success of your treatment. Whatever position you choose it is vital that it affords complete relaxation for both you and the receiver.

A professional reflexologist will undoubtedly have a massage couch. It is not essential for you to purchase one although you may decide to invest in one later on.

You may decide to work with the receiver lying on a bed. You would need to place pillows/ cushions under the head to support the neck and also to enable you to observe any facial expressions. Pillows/cushions can also be placed under the receiver's knees for comfort and it is a good idea to place a cushion under the hand you are about to treat. This provides a comfortable working position for you to work from. You will sit to one side facing the receiver. Towels or blankets are essential to cover up the receiver. This not only makes the receiver feel safe and secure but it also counteracts the loss of body heat, which will occur as the treatment progresses.

You may prefer to work on the floor and this is also acceptable. You will need a well-padded surface which can be made by placing a thick duvet, some blankets or sleeping bags on the floor. As before, for the receiver's comfort place pillows under the head and under the knees and cover them up. Put a cushion under your knees for your own comfort and a cushion under the hand which you are treating first.

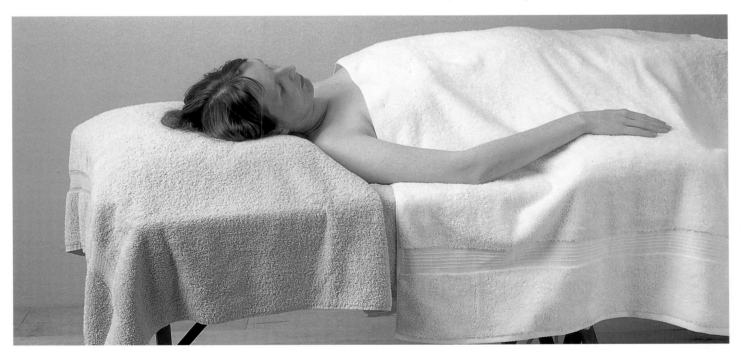

If using a couch or bed, ensure the receiver is warm and comfortable.

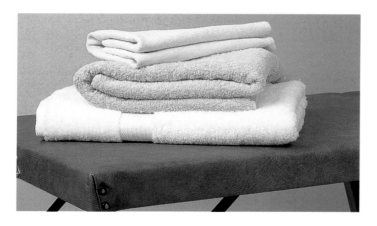

A supply of towels is essential to ensure the receiver stays warm and relaxed.

Some reflexologists work with the receiver sitting on a chair with their hand resting on a stool or table at the side but this position is potentially not as comfortable and seems to encourage conversation which is not conducive to complete relaxation.

Another possibility, is to sit facing the receiver with his/her hand resting on a cushion on a table or bench.

OTHER POINTS TO REMEMBER:

- Have extra towels/blankets on hand just in case the receiver feels cold.
- Remove all jewellery from your hands to avoid scratching.
- Ask the receiver to remove his/her jewellery so that the treatment is not impeded.
- Any restrictive clothing such as ties and belts may be loosened to maximise comfort.
- Clip your nails closely to avoid digging them in.
- Check your nails are clean!
- Wash your hands prior to a treatment.
- Do not use oils or creams during the reflexology session. Lubricants make it difficult to hold the hands properly, cause your fingers and thumbs to slip and decrease your sensitivity. You may use them at the end of the reflexology sequence.

Facing the receiver across a table or bench is a simple and effective reflexology position.

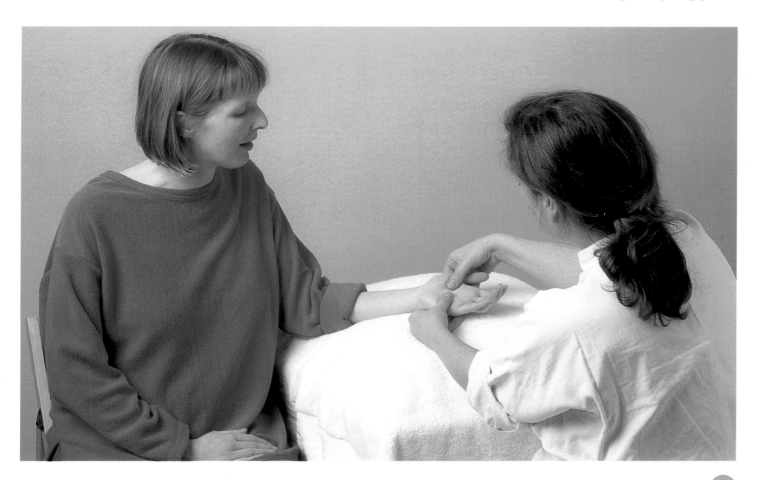

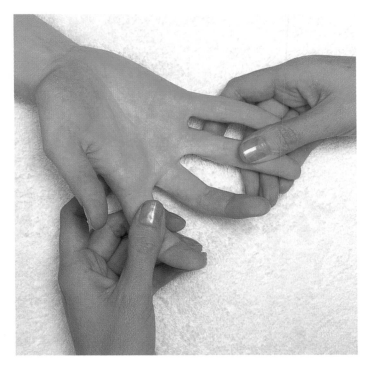

A visual examination of the hands is essential before starting a treatment.

EXAMINING THE HANDS

Prior to starting your treatment it is very enlightening to examine the hands visually. You will be amazed at what the hands can reveal. A healthy person will have hands that are a good colour with unblemished skin and good muscle tone. The hands should feel pleasantly warm but not excessively moist and clammy. Nails should have a strong and healthy appearance. Here are some points to observe:

- Infections of the hands and nails
- Calluses and hard skin
- Thin skin
- Blisters
- Cracks and crevices
- Warts
- Scars
- Cuts
- Spots and rashes
- Colour – too pale, too red, yellow, purple or mottled.

- Nails – split, flaked, broken. Are they hardened, thickened, ridged, spotted or a peculiar shape? (Spoon-shaped nails are sometimes seen in iron-deficiency anaemia)
- Shape of the fingers and thumbs – are they bent or straight and or puffy?

Any of these abnormalities indicate an imbalance of a reflex zone or zones. It is not relevant what the abnormality is—what is important is the SITE. For instance if there is a wart or some hard skin located on the outer aspect of the thumb this could indicate that there is a neck problem.

Puffiness around the wrist would indicate an imbalance of the lymphatic system as the pelvic lymphatic reflex area is located around the wrist.

You will now look at your hands in a new light.

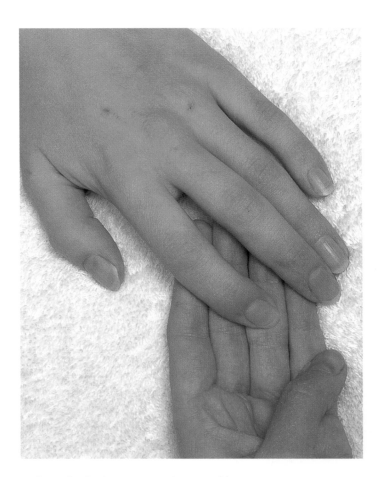

A deviated index finger may signify sinus problems.

CONTRA-INDICATIONS TO HAND REFLEXOLOGY

Although reflexology is a very safe form of therapy there are some occasions when a treatment is not advisable or care should be taken.

- For any serious condition being treated by a medical practitioner. The receiver should check with the doctor that reflexology is acceptable – it usually is

- Fevers – this shows that the body is fighting off toxins. A reflexology treatment may release more toxins into the system. Wait until the fever has subsided

- Contagious skin diseases such as scabies – you do not want to spread it or catch it yourself! (NB conditions like eczema and psoriasis are NOT contagious)

- Deep vein thrombosis or phlebitis – a clot could move

- After surgery – research shows that reflexology can help the body to recover more quickly but only a light treatment is given for the first few weeks after surgery

- Pregnancy – hand reflexology is not recommended for the first three months where there is a history of miscarriage

- Avoid cuts, scars, bruises, wounds, severe varicose veins or any other areas which are painful to the touch

- Corns and calluses – use gentle pressure if they are tender

- Take care over the pancreas reflex when treating a diabetic

- Use less pressure when treating a diabetic as the skin may be thinner, more fragile, bruises easily and can heal more slowly

- Elderly – use lighter treatments generally as the skin tends to be thinner and osteoporosis (fragile bones) or arthritis in the hands may be present

- Children require a light pressure – the younger they are the less time they require

- Terminally ill – use a gentle pressure

- Heart area – take care over the heart reflex if there are cardiac problems

- Take care are not to apply strong pressure – a treatment should not be painful

- Do not over-treat one particular area

- Do not diagnose, make claims or promise cures

POSSIBLE REACTIONS TO HAND REFLEXOLOGY

Following a treatment it is quite normal to get a response. Both physical and psychological changes may occur – this is excellent and shows that your treatment is really working.

Below is a list of reactions, which have occurred after treatments showing that a positive effect has been achieved.

REMEMBER ONLY ONE OR TWO REACTIONS MAY OCCUR AND SHOULD DISAPPEAR WITHIN 24 HOURS

- A state of deep relaxation and a sense of euphoria

- A warm glow as energy blockages are released

- Frequent dreaming

- Deeper sleep

- Emotional changes as emotions are released

- Rashes, pimples and increased perspiration as the activity of the skin is increased

- More frequent urination – sometimes the urine may be cloudy or smelly

- Bowels move more frequently and volume of the stools may increase

- Runny nose

- Coughing as mucus is expelled

- Colds and sore throats

- Watery eyes

- Fever

- Previous illnesses, which have been suppressed, may flare up temporarily and then disappear

- Vaginal discharges

- Toothache

- A need to drink more water to flush away the toxins

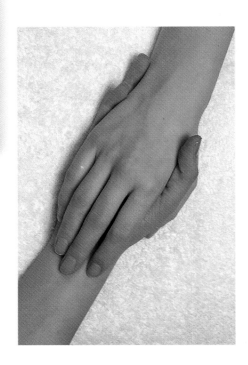

hand relaxation
Techniques

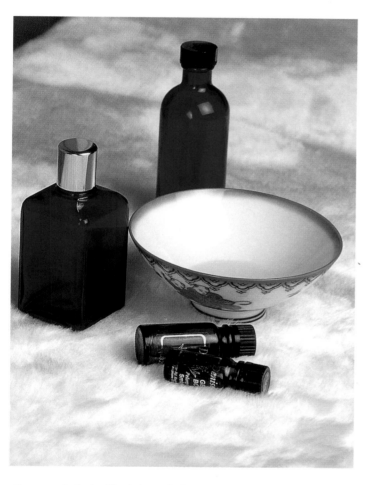

Creams and oils should only be used after treatment.

The first contact between your hands and the receiver's hands is so important. The relaxation techniques will help to put both of you at ease and build up a sense of trust.

You will find that it will feel very natural to you to work on someone's hands and any initial nervousness and hesitation will disappear. These techniques will be enjoyable for both of you.

As your confidence grows do be creative and develop your own new techniques. Any movements that feel good to you will feel wonderful to the receiver.

Relaxation techniques should always begin and end a hand reflexology treatment. You will need to spend about ten minutes at the beginning of a session and a few minutes at the end. You can also include a few during your reflexology procedure.

Perform all the relaxation techniques on one hand before moving onto the other hand.

Ideally no creams or oils should be used for your preliminary relaxation sequence otherwise when you try to carry out the reflexology procedure the hands will be too slippery to apply sufficient pressure to the reflexology points. However, at the end of the treatment a small amount of oil or cream can be used. If the hands do feel at all greasy at the end of the relaxation session then just wipe them gently with a towel.

If you do not have time to give a hand reflexology treatment then this relaxation routine on its own can be very beneficial. Our hands are in constant use throughout the day and they really appreciate a massage! Massage them everyday with creams or oil to thoroughly moisturise the skin and keep them soft and smooth. A hand massage can be given any time, any place, anywhere. Before you start remember to remove all watches and jewellery.

GREETING THE HANDS

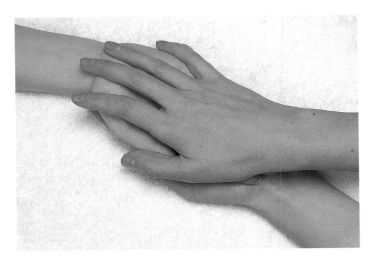

This initial contact will help to relax and reassure the receiver. Take hold of the receiver's right hand between both of your hands and gently clasp it for a few minutes. Work with your eyes closed to heighten your sensitivity. Try to become aware of any tension and imagine it flowing out through your hands.

STROKING THE HANDS AND LOWER ARM

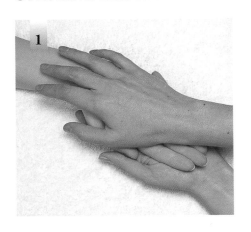

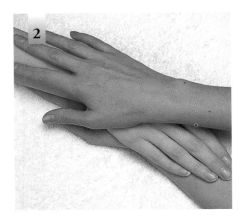

Support the forearm with your left hand and gently stroke up the hand and arm with your right hand (1). As you reach the elbow glide lightly back with no pressure down the arm and hand (2). The receiver will experience a deep sense of well-being and relaxation as the nerves are soothed and the tension melts away. You will feel the hand warm up as you help to stimulate the circulation and aid the elimination of toxins.

STROKING THE HANDS

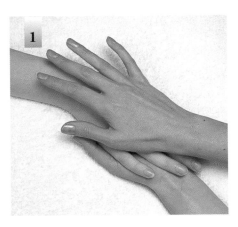

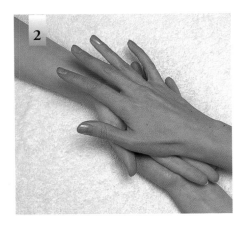

Supporting their right wrist with your left hand, stroke up to the top of the hand only. Repeat this movement several times. (1)

Now turn their hand over and repeat on the palm of their hand. (2)

For a deeper movement, stroke the palm with the heel of your hand.

OPENING THE HANDS – I

Take the right hand in both of yours with the palm uppermost. Start at the wrist with your thumbs parallel and touching in the centre of the palm. (1)

Slide your thumbs out to the side gently opening up the palm of the hand. Repeat this movement in rows until you reach the base of the fingers. (2)

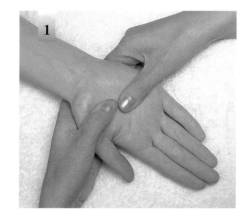
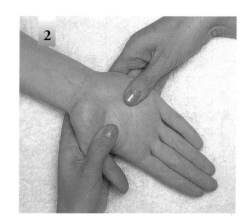

OPENING THE HANDS – II

Turn the hand over and repeat the movements above on the top of the hand.

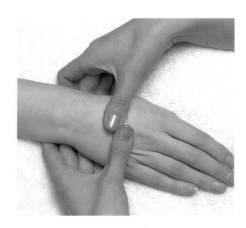
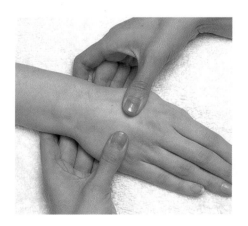

WORKING THE PALM OF THE HAND

With the palm uppermost interlock your little fingers with the receiver's right hand – one with the little finger, one with the thumb. (1)

Bring your thumbs round onto the palm and work into the palm with small round outward circular movements. (2)

You can work quite firmly into the palm of the hand. If your own hands are not very flexible then try the next technique.

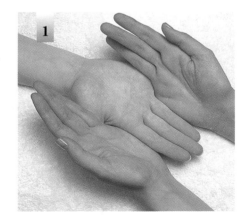
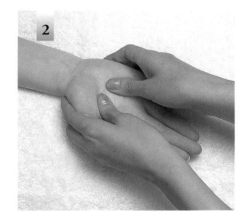

KNUCKLING THE PALM OF THE HAND

Make a fist with your right hand and support the receiver's hand, palm uppermost, with your other hand. Work into the palm of their hand with circular movements using your knuckles. This movement helps to loosen muscles, joints and tendons. It also increases the flexibility of your own hands.

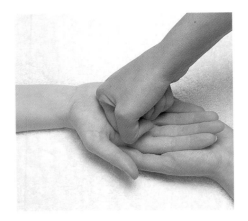
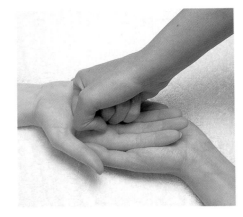

STROKING BETWEEN THE BONES

Hold the receiver's hand with one hand to give support. Use the thumb of your free hand to work along each of the furrows between the bones of the hand. Start between the knuckles and stroke down towards the wrist.(1)

Now use your index finger to perform the same movement. (2)

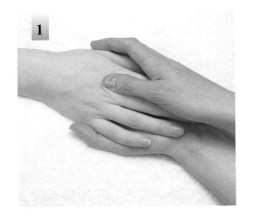
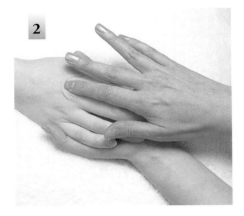

LOOSENING THE WRIST

Support the hand with your fingers. Use your thumbs to work in small circles all around the inside of the wrist. (1)

Now turn the hand over and work in the same way on the other side of the wrist.(2)

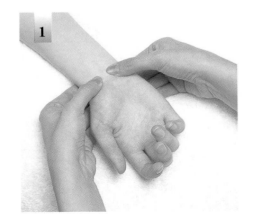
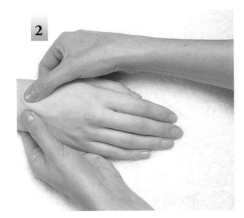

MOVING THE WRIST

Interlock your fingers with the receiver and then bend the wrist
SLOWLY and GENTLY, first forwards (1) and backwards. (2)

Then bend the wrist from side to side. (3)

Finally, rotate clockwise and anti-clockwise (4)

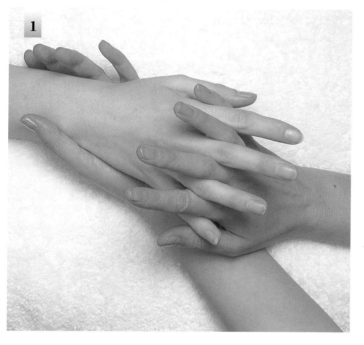

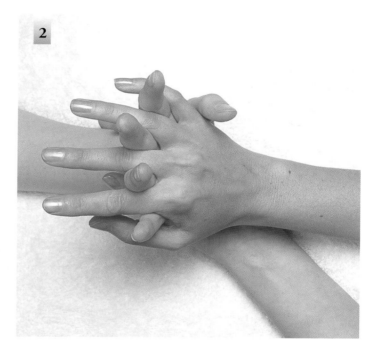

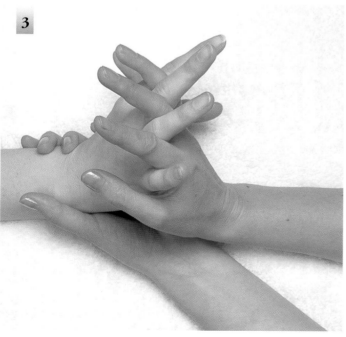

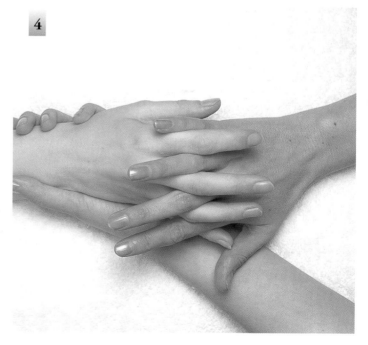

WRIST ROLLING

This technique is really invigorating. Leave the upper arm down on the couch and lift up the forearm. Place your palms on the sides of the receiver's wrist. Move your hands rapidly back and forth. The receiver's hand should flop and move loosely as you perform this movement.(1)

If you prefer you may slot your thumbs in between the thumbs and little finger to perform this movement. (2)

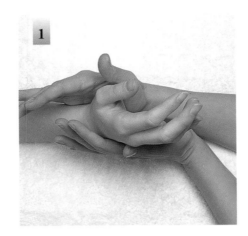
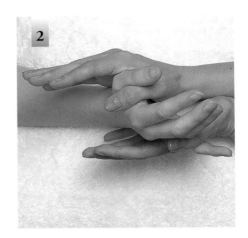

STRETCH AND SQUEEZE THE FINGERS AND THUMB

Hold the receiver's wrist to support the hand. Gently and slowly stretch and squeeze each finger individually working from the knuckle to the tip.

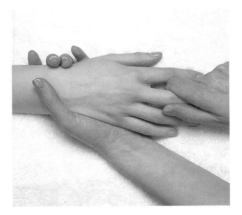
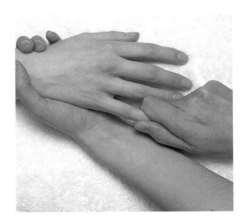

LOOSEN THE FINGERS AND THUMB

Make circular pressures around each joint using your thumb and index finger.

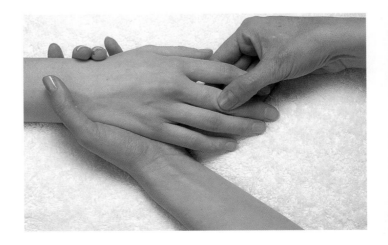

BENDING THE FINGERS AND THUMB

Gently flex and extend each finger and thumb joint with your thumb and index finger. (There are 2 joints in the thumb, 3 in the fingers).

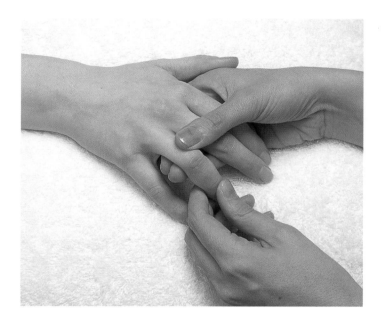 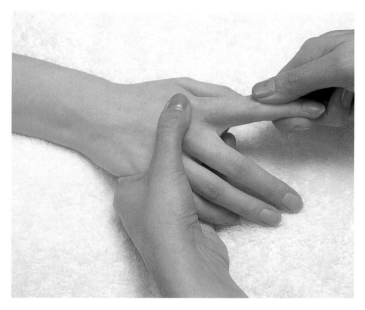

CIRCLING

Circle the thumb and fingers individually both clockwise (1) and anti-clockwise. (2)

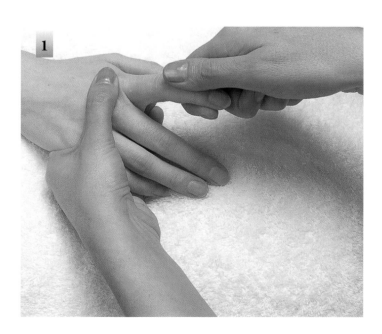 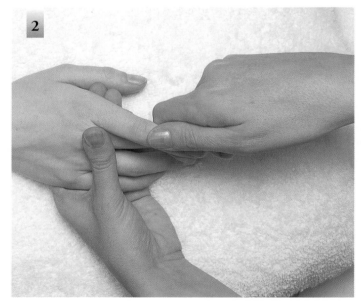

SOLAR PLEXUS RELEASE

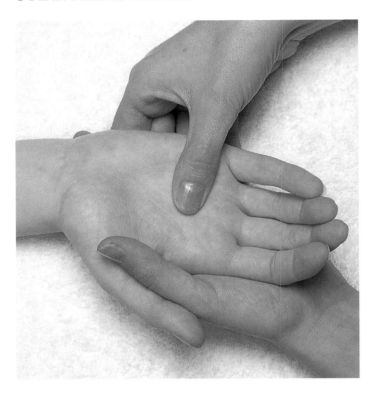

To release any remaining tension place your thumb on the solar plexus reflex which is found almost in the centre of the palm and press slowly and gently into it.

FINGERTIP STROKING

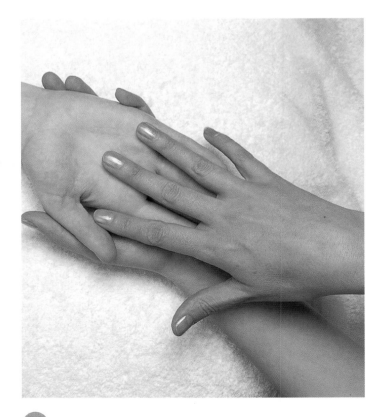

To end your relaxation routine sandwich the receiver's hand between your palm and using your fingertips stroke the hand slowly from the wrist to the tips.

Now practice all these relaxation techniques on the other hand.

basic hand reflexology
Techniques

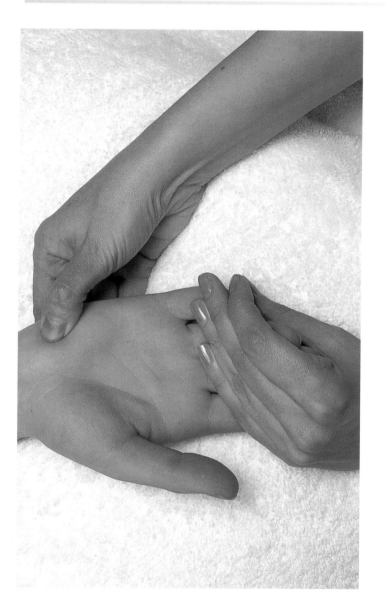

Now that you have mastered the relaxation techniques, you are going to learn how to treat the reflex areas in the hand. The reflex points are tiny and the thumb is the main tool used for applying pressure although on certain areas of the hand the fingers are used.

Please note the following before you begin:

1) Keep fingernails short – a nail digging into the skin is very painful.

2) You and the receiver should remove all watches, bracelets and rings.

3) Use only the flat pads of your fingers and thumbs to prevent even short nails from scratching or digging in.

4) Do not apply too much pressure – reflexology should not be uncomfortable.

5) Do not use oil or cream on the receiver's hands for the preliminary relaxation movements or for the step by step procedure. If the hands are sticky or slippery then you will not be able to make good contact with the reflex points. Oils also decrease your sensitivity making it difficult for you to pinpoint any abnormal areas. Oils and creams may be used for the final relaxation movements.

HOLDING TECHNIQUE

It is very important to support the hands properly during the treatment so that you have full control and exude an air of confidence. You also need to be able to reach and pinpoint the reflex zones easily and effectively.

Never grip the hand that you are working on too tightly or pull the skin taut otherwise the receiver will feel tense and uncomfortable.

Remember to place a pillow or cushion under the receiver's hand, which should be covered with a towel to protect it if you are intending to use oils at the end of the session.

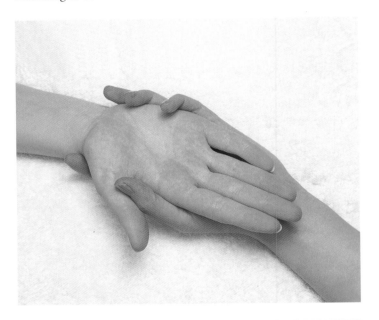

For most of the treatment the receiver's hand, palm uppermost, will be cupped in the palm of your hand with your thumb steadying on the palmar side.

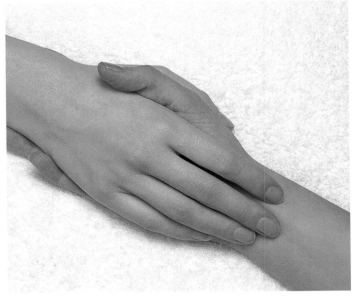

If you are working on the top (dorsal side), hold the hand by supporting the wrist from underneath in a 'handshake' position.

THUMB WALKING/CATERPILLAR WALKING TECHNIQUE

This technique is used for working large areas of the hand. Place the flat pad part of your thumb on the area to be treated and then bend the first joint SLIGHTLY and then unbend the thumb slightly so that you move forward a little.

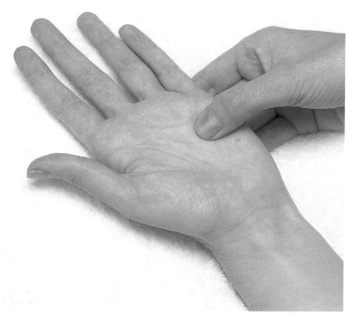

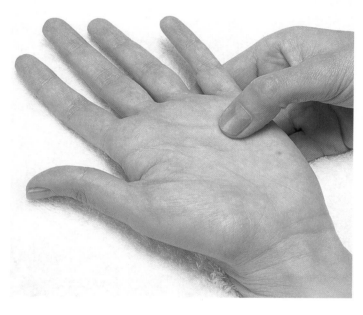

Continue in this way moving forward in tiny creeping movements like a caterpillar without losing contact with the hand. It is impossible to walk with a straight thumb and if you bend the thumb too much your nail will dig into the skin. Try this technique on the palm of your own hand.

Whilst your thumb is walking your other fingers should rest gently around the hand. Try to maintain a constant and even pressure always working in a forward direction. Do not worry if your movements feel somewhat jerky and clumsy at first. Persevere and you will achieve a smooth, consistent pressure.

REMEMBER

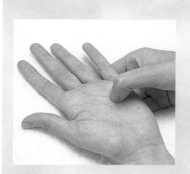

Thumb too arched (incorrect)

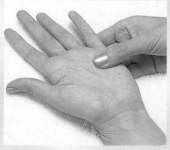

Thumb too flat (incorrect)

- Do not dig in with your nails
- Bend only the first joint of the thumb
- Bend the thumb slightly – it should be neither too bent nor too straight
- Take very small steps
- Movements are always forwards never backwards
- Pressure should be steady
- Pressure should be firm yet not hard enough to induce pain

PRESSURE CIRCLES

Pressure circles may be performed with the pad of the thumb or a finger. They can be used for working specific reflex points or to relieve the sensitivity of tender reflexes.

Place your thumb or finger on to a reflex point and press gently into the area. Keeping this pressure constant, circle gently over the point several times.

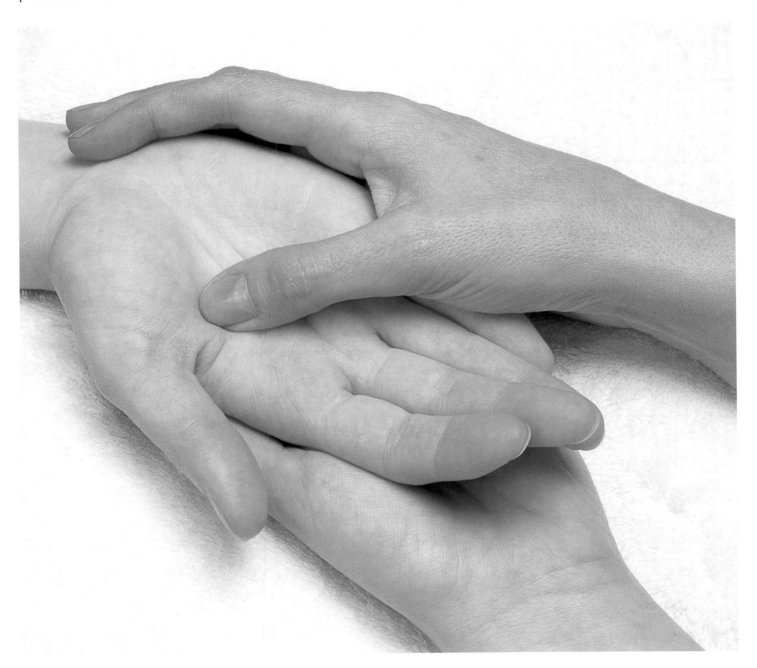

Pressure circles on the kidney point.

FINGER WALKING

The finger walking technique is almost the same as thumb walking. The object is the same—to exert a constant steady pressure, which is comfortable and effective for the receiver. Use finger walking in preference to thumb walking on bony or sensitive areas such as the top surface of the hand.

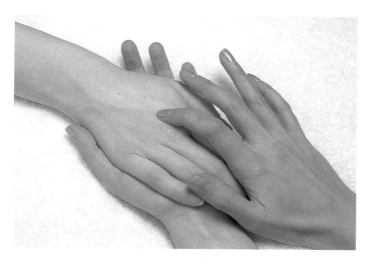

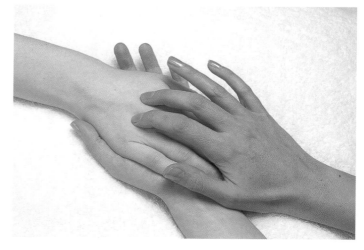

Practice SINGLE finger walking first. Place the tip of your index finger on the area to be treated. Bend the first joint of the finger slightly and then unbend it a little to move the fingertip in a forward direction. Try this technique on the back of the hand, walking from the knuckles towards your wrist and remember to take the smallest possible steps.

Now try MULTIPLE finger walking using two or more fingers, once again working down the top surface of the hand.

If you are working on top of the hand walking downwards, place your fist under the palm of the hand to support it. Practice with one, two or three fingers to see which is most comfortable for you and the receiver.

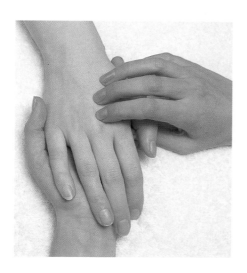

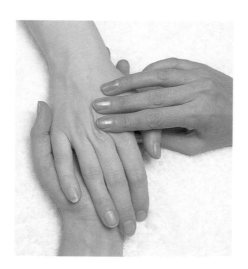

REMEMBER

- Maintain a steady even pressure

- Move only in a forward direction

- Take care not to dig your nails in

- Take only very small steps

- Use very gentle pressure — finger walking is specifically designed for bony and sensitive areas

You may also work sideways across the top (dorsal surface) of the hand. When working sideways your thumb will be placed under the palm of the hand to support it while your fingers walk across the top.

PRESS AND RELEASE

This technique is particularly effective for relieving pain and you may perform it with either your thumb or finger. Press into a tender point for about several seconds (here the ovary is illustrated).

Release the pressure and repeat several times until the sensitivity decreases.

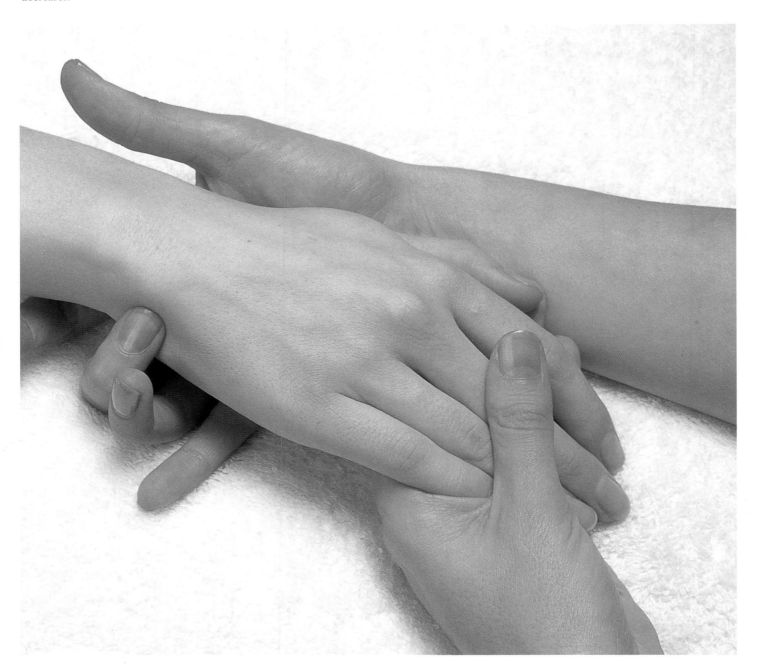

Press and release on the ovary area.

ROTATION ON A POINT

This technique involves pinpointing an area to be treated and rotating the hand around it. Thus the term–'rotating on a point'. Place the pad of your thumb or finger on the relevant reflex point. (Here the right ovary is illustrated).

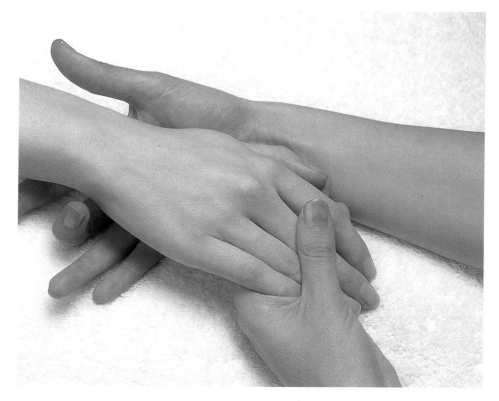

Use your other hand to rotate the receiver's hand around the point several times.

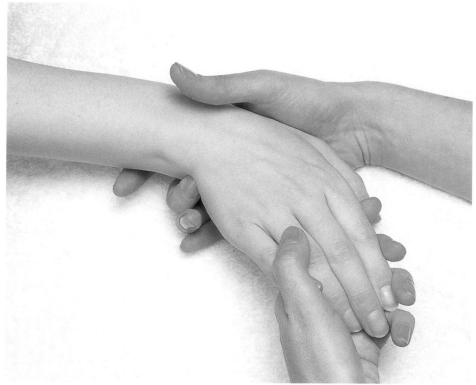

Hook in and Back-up

To access specific points requiring greater accuracy, this technique is excellent. It would never be used for covering a large area— thumb or finger walking would be much more appropriate.

Press your thumb into your chosen point and apply pressure (hook in) and then pull back across the point (back-up).

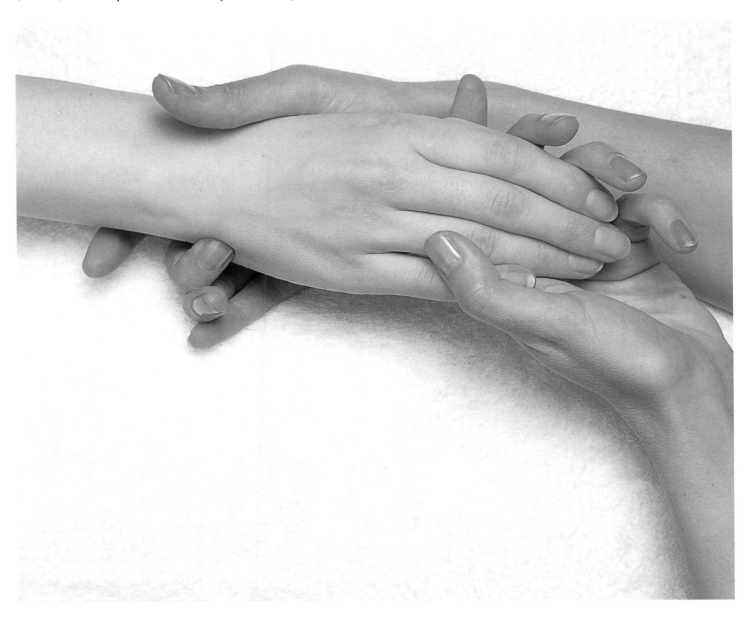

beginning a hand reflexology
Treatment

This section of the book will guide you step-by-step through a complete hand reflexology routine. Colour photographs and detailed instructions demonstrate very clearly how to perform the treatment. At the end of each step there are guidelines explaining which conditions would respond favourably to treatment of that particular reflex area.

Please study the following diagram to familiarise yourself with the different surfaces of the hands. The last section of the book

contains hand charts, which indicate the position of every reflex area.

You are going to treat the whole of the right hand before we move on to the left hand. It is very confusing to swap from one hand to the other when you are learning and the continuity of the treatment is destroyed every time you break contact.

Surfaces of the hands

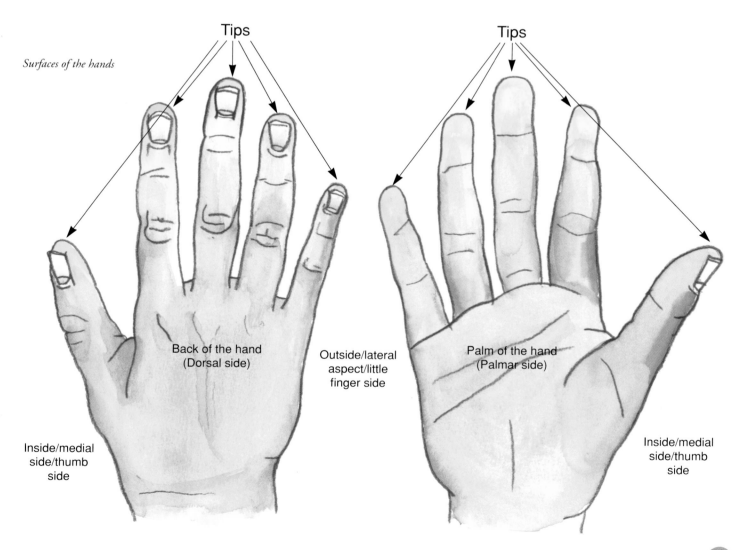

Tips

Tips

Back of the hand
(Dorsal side)

Outside/lateral
aspect/little
finger side

Palm of the hand
(Palmar side)

Inside/medial
side/thumb
side

Inside/medial
side/thumb
side

HOW MUCH PRESSURE TO USE

The amount of pressure you exert should be adjusted to the person who you are treating. It varies enormously from one individual to another. Some hands are incredibly sensitive whereas others appear to show no reaction. Physical people tend to prefer a firmer touch whereas more spiritual souls usually favour a very gentle less physical treatment. Very deep pressure is not helpful and will result in the receiver jerking his/her hand away from you in pain. Reflexology should never be painful.

Never assume that a person will always require the same amount of pressure. Hands often become sensitised when a person is highly stressed after an emotional trauma or very debilitated. Painkillers and other medications that de-sensitise feeling will of course make the reflexes less sensitive.

In general expect to use more pressure on a young healthy adult than a frail or elderly person or a child. If you discover any tender reflexes then perform gentle pressure circles over the area without causing undue discomfort to the receiver. Treatment should NEVER be applied continuously over one reflex point. It is much more effective to return to any sensitive areas at frequent intervals and more comfortable.

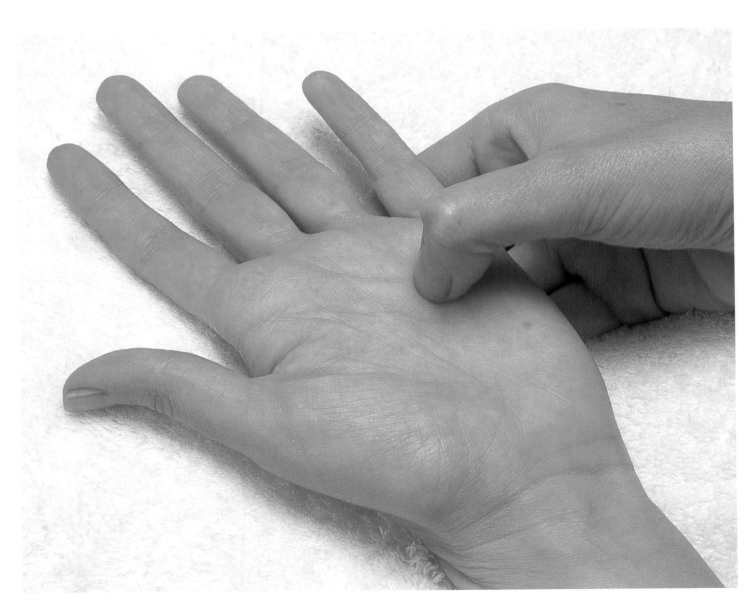

Maintain a firm but gentle pressure. Very deep pressure can be painful.

HOW LONG TO SPEND ON A TREATMENT

A complete hand reflexology treatment (with practice) will probably take you about 40 minutes. If you are working on a child, a frail elderly person or the very sick then 20 minutes will probably be sufficient. A baby would only need a five minute treatment consisting mainly of stroking movements using a feather-like touch followed by light pressure on the reflex areas showing symptoms.

Do not assume that longer is better. If the session is too lengthy this can result in over-stimulation of the body and excessive elimination.

HOW OFTEN TO TREAT

For optimum results carry out the complete hand reflexology routine once a week for about 6-8 treatments. This gives the body plenty of time for self-healing in between treatments. It is possible that a minor reaction will occur after a session, which should pass within 24 hours.

If there is an acute problem such as a sore throat then the reflex area to the throat and other areas of sensitivity can be treated at least once a day until the symptoms subside.

After the initial sessions a treatment once every 2-4 weeks will help to maintain health and prevent problems from occurring. Of course if you wish to pamper the receiver then once a week is quite acceptable.

WHAT THE RECEIVER WILL FEEL

Generally a sense of incredible relaxation and tranquillity is experienced during a treatment. The alpha state of relaxation is generated during a reflexology session which is a level of consciousness at which healing can take place. Some people feel tingling sensations or warmth as blockages are released and others experience a sharp sensation or a dull ache where a reflex area is congested. Everyone is so different. The receiver will awake refreshed and restored with a wonderful sense of well-being.

VISUAL EXAMINATION

After you have made both yourself and the receiver comfortable, examine the hands for any hard skin, cracks, warts, bruises, problematic nails etc. Remember to work gently over tender areas.

Make sure that your body is totally relaxed, particularly your neck and shoulders and that your mind is calm and peaceful. You will begin with the right hand.

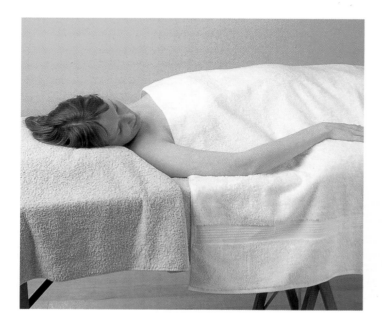

Particularly if using a bed or a couch, a reflexology treatment is extremely relaxing.

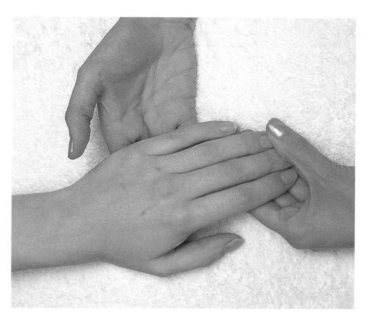

Always check hands for tender areas such as bruises or cuts.

Right Hand

RELAXATION TECHNIQUES

Please refer back to the relevant chapter for a full description of all of the relaxation techniques. The following are simply suggestions – feel free to choose your favourites.

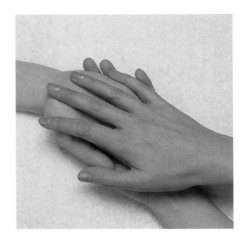

Greeting the hand

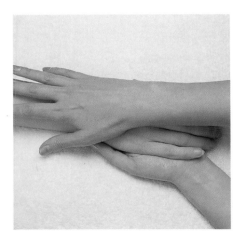

Stroking the hand and lower arm

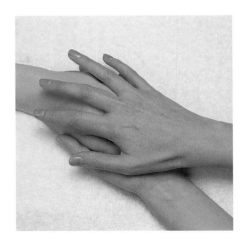

Stroking the hand – palm down

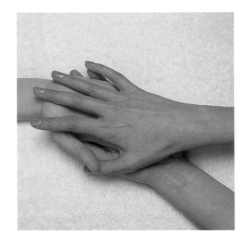

Stroking the hand – palm up

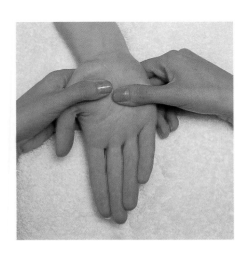

Opening the hand – palm up

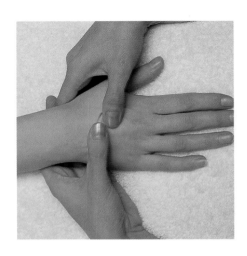

Opening the hand – palm down

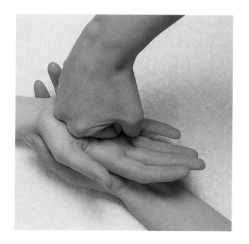

Knuckling the palm

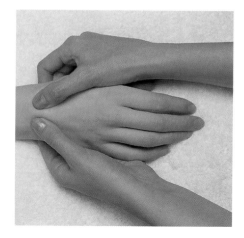

Loosening the wrist

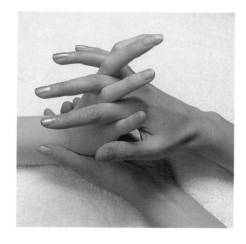

Moving the wrist forward and backward

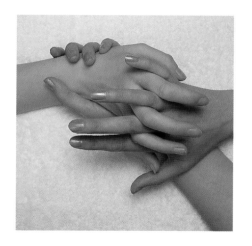

Rotating the wrist

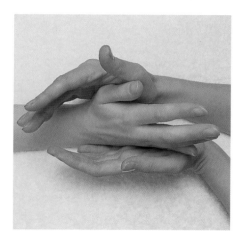

Wrist rolling

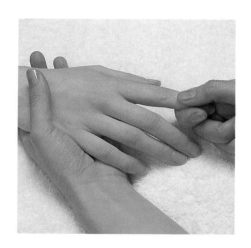

Loosening the fingers and thumb

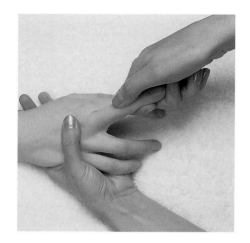

Moving the fingers

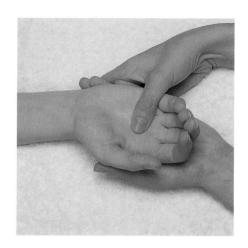

Solar plexus release

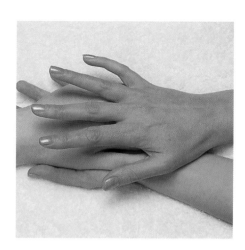

Fingertip stroking

HEAD AND NECK AREA

STEP 1 – HEAD AND BRAIN (BACK AND SIDES OF THE THUMB)

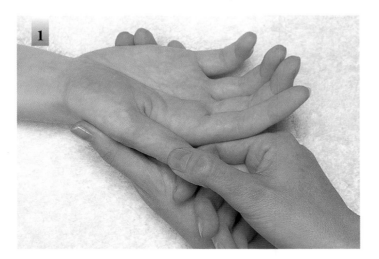

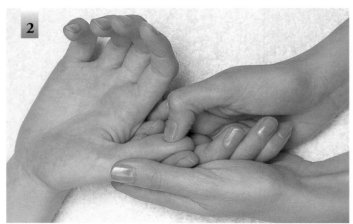

Start with the receiver's right palm uppermost. Use your right thumb to walk from the very tip of the thumb in parallel lines down the outside (1), the back (2) and the inside (3).

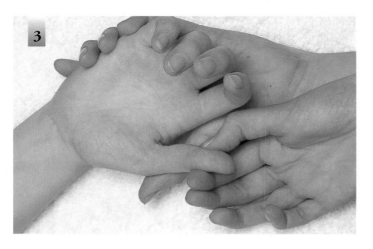

USES: Headaches and migraine. Any problems involving the brain, e.g. Parkinson's disease, Alzheimer's disease, stroke, lack of concentration, poor memory, cerebral palsy, multiple sclerosis and dyslexia. It is also effective for lessening the after effects of an anaesthetic.

STEP 2 – PITUITARY GLAND (CENTRE OF THE BACK OF THE THUMB)

The pituitary gland is located roughly in the centre of the fleshy part of the thumb. Often it is slightly off-centre – higher, lower, more to the left or to the right – so be prepared to search for this point. Support the thumb with the fingers of your left hand and use the hook in and back-up technique with your right thumb to treat the pituitary gland.

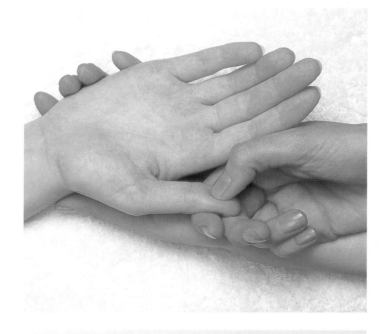

USES: All hormonal problems such as pre-menstrual syndrome and the menopause.
Any problems with the reproductive organs. Thyroid problems.

STEP 3 – FACE (FRONT OF THE THUMB)

Turn the hand over. Walk down the front of the thumb from the tip of the thumb to the base using your thumb or index finger. Caterpillar walk down as many times as necessary to cover the entire area – it depends how big the thumb is.

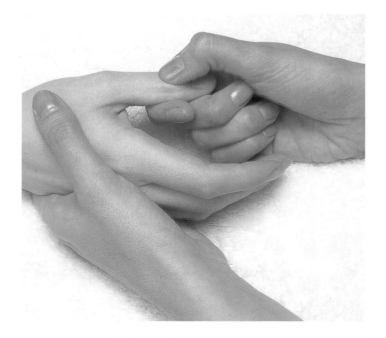

USES: Any problems involving the face including eye, nose, sinus, teeth, lips, gums, mouth and jaw problems.
This area is particularly effective for alleviating the excruciating pain of facial neuralgia and for Bell's palsy (facial paralysis).

STEP 4 – NECK ROTATION (BASE OF THE THUMB)

Grasp the thumb between your index finger and thumb and rotate it clockwise and anti-clockwise. This is like rotating the neck. If the joint creaks or is limited in movement this reflects a neck problem.

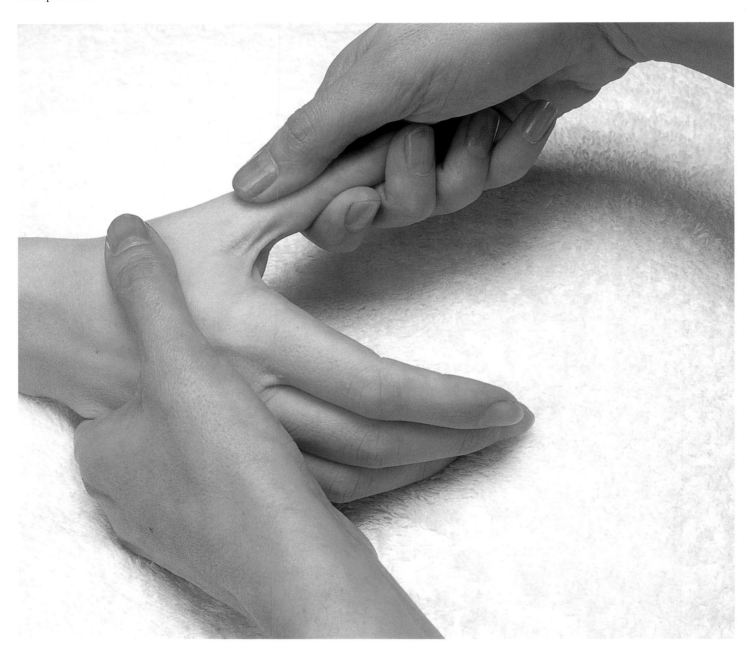

USES: Neck pain, lack of mobility in the neck, whiplash injuries

STEP 5 – NECK/THYROID (BACK AND FRONT OF THE BASE OF THE THUMB)

Wrap your hand around the receiver's hand with your thumb across the palmar side of the tip of the thumb, fingers around the top of the hand. Thumb walk across the base of the back of the thumb.

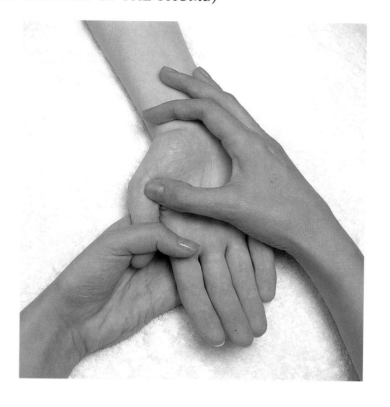

Now turn the hand over and grasp the thumb between your left thumb and index finger. Thumb walk across the base of the front of the thumb with your right thumb.

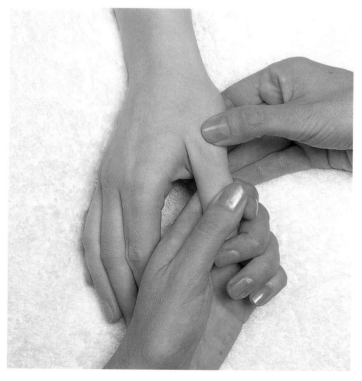

USES: All neck problems, disorders of the throat, tonsils and vocal cords, thyroid and parathyroid.

STEP 6 – SINUSES (BACK, SIDES AND TOP OF THE FINGERS)

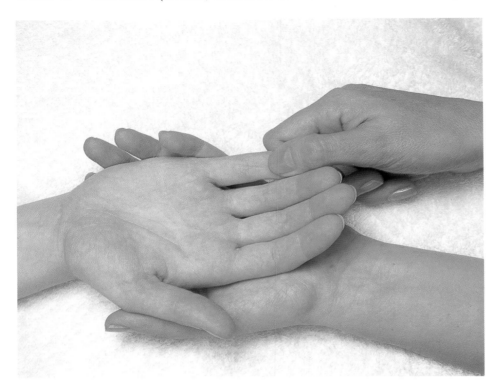

Cradle the receiver's right hand in the palm of your left hand, palm uppermost. Start from the top of the little finger and with your right thumb work down to the base of the little finger. About four rows of thumb walking will cover the area thoroughly.

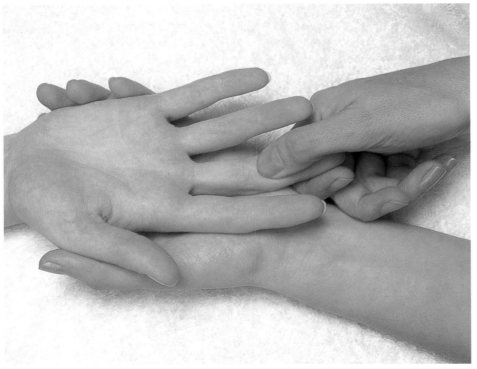

Repeat on the ring, middle and index finger. (Here the middle finger is shown).

USES: Sinus problems, hay fever, catarrh, allergies and colds.

STEP 7 – TEETH (DORSAL SIDE OF THE FINGERS)

Turn the hand over to work the front of the fingers. Start at the
tip of the index finger and do about three rows of finger walking
in parallel lines to completely cover each finger.

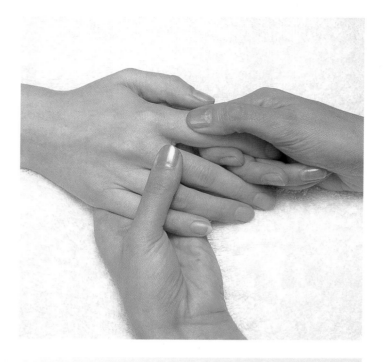

USES: Toothache; sensitive, infected or painful gums; abscesses.

STEP 8 – UPPER LYMPHATICS (WEBBING OF THE FINGERS)

With the top of the hand uppermost, use your thumb and index
finger to gently squeeze in between each of the fingers.

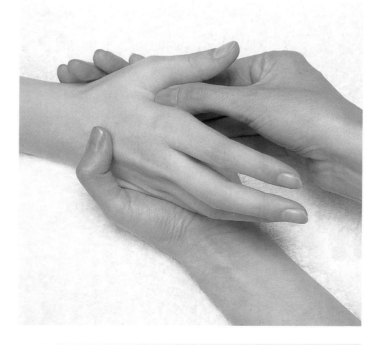

USES: To drain the head and neck, to fight off infection and boost the immune system.

STEP 9 – SPINE/SCIATIC LINE (INSIDE EDGE OF THE HAND/THE WRIST)

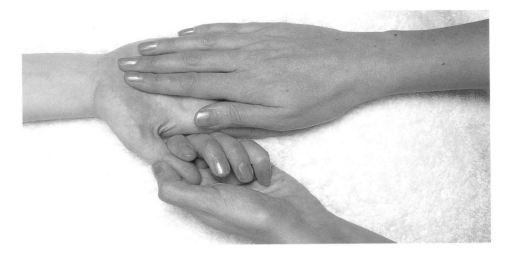

The cervical (neck) area of the spine is found between the first and second joints of the thumb and as you work down the inside edge of the hand you are covering the thoracic area (mid-back) and lumbar area (low back).

Place your right hand palm down on top of the receiver's hand, which should be palm uppermost. Start at the neck area.

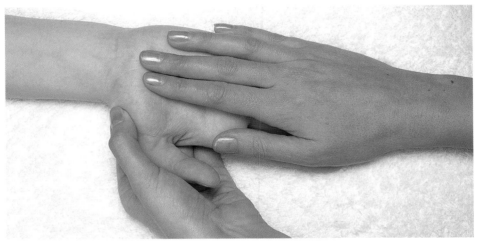

Then walk your left thumb down the inside of the hand.

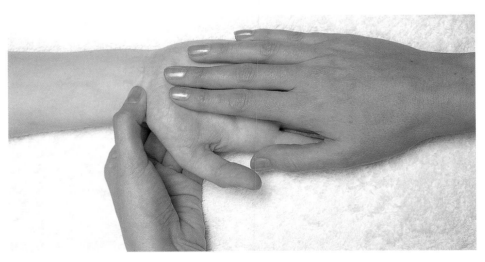

Continue to walk across the wrist until you reach the other side of the hand to cover the sciatic area.

USES: All back disorders including general aches and pains, degeneration of the spine, disc problems and sciatica.

STEP 10 – RIGHT EYE AND EAR. (BASE OF THE FINGERS)

Clasp the right hand in your left hand, fingers underneath, thumb across the receiver's fingers to hold them gently back. With your right thumb walk across the ridge at the base of the fingers working from the little finger to the index finger. Walk slowly across the area again. Stop between fingers 4 and 5, which is the ear point. Press and release.

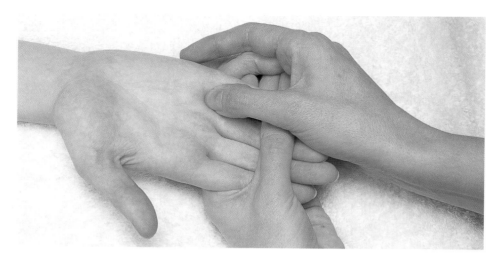

Continue to thumb walk, stopping between fingers 3 and 4, the eustachian tube. Press and release.

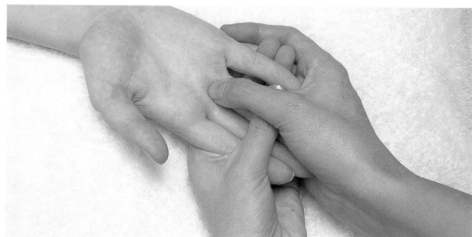

To complete the eye/ear area walk to between the index and middle finger – the eye point. Press and release.

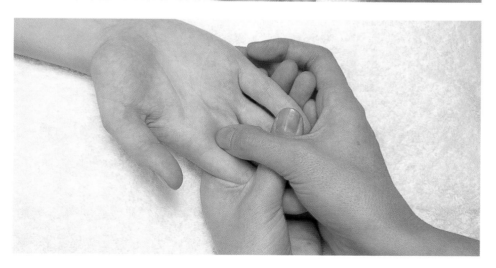

USES: All conditions involving the eyes including sore, tired or watery eyes, blocked tear ducts, glaucoma, cataracts and conjunctivitis. Ear problems such as ear infections, glue ear, tinnitus, vertigo and dizziness.

STEP 11 – RIGHT LUNG/CHEST (PALM OF HAND)

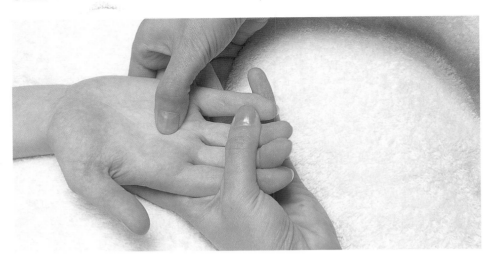

Support the hand palm uppermost with your left hand and thumb walk in horizontal strips across the hand with your thumb, starting from the base of the little fingers until you reach the diaphragm line.

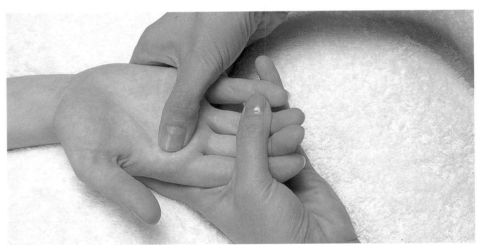

If you find any 'gritty' areas indicating congestion then do some pressure circles to gently disperse the crystals.

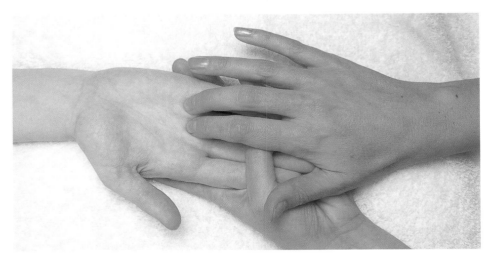

If you prefer you may caterpillar walk in vertical strips using one or more fingers.

USES: All respiratory problems including chesty coughs, asthma, bronchitis, emphysema, pleurisy, hyperventilation and panic attacks.

STEP 12 – RIGHT LUNG/BREAST/MAMMARY GLANDS (TOP OF HAND)

Turn the hand over. To work on the top of the hand grasp the fingers with your left hand, thumb on top, fingers underneath and use your right index finger to walk down the hand in vertical strips working from the base of the fingers to the diaphragm line.

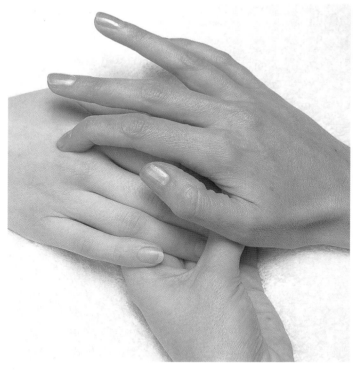

If you wish you may work across the hand from the base of the index finger towards the little finger. This area occupies approximately the upper third of the top of the hand.

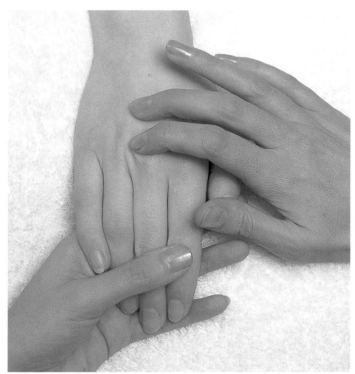

USES: All respiratory problems as described in Step 11. Also breast problems such as soreness due to pre-menstrual syndrome.

STEP 13 – LIVER/GALLBLADDER (RIGHT HAND ONLY)

The liver is found predominantly in zones 3, 4 and 5 between the diaphragm line and the waistline. Supporting the palm uppermost with your left hand use your right thumb to work from zone 5 (little finger side) to zone 3 across the palm of the hand.

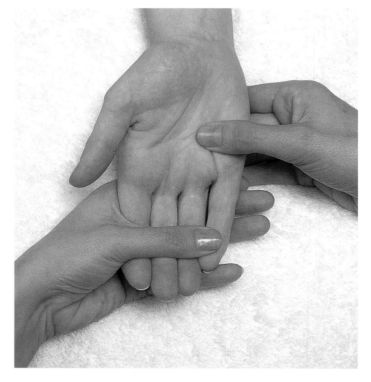

The gallbladder reflex lies within the region of the liver usually in line with the fourth finger. Probe the area and you may feel a slight indentation, which represents the reflex area of the gallbladder. Use the hook in and back-up technique or pressure circles to treat this area.

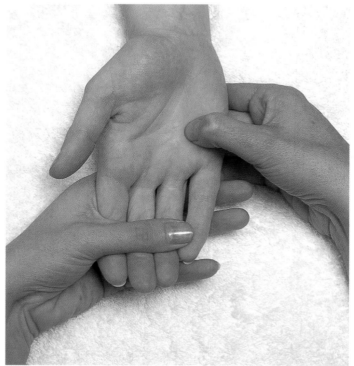

USES: All digestive conditions especially nausea, jaundice, problems with fat digestion and detoxification.

STEP 14 – STOMACH/PANCREAS/DUODENUM

Supporting with your right hand, use your left thumb to work the remaining area in horizontal rows between the diaphragm line and waistline. Two to three rows should cover this area.

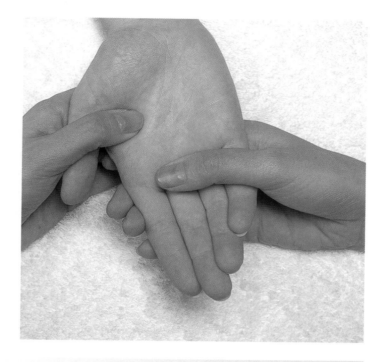

USES: Stomach problems including indigestion, hyperacidity, ulcers, general digestive disorders and diabetes.

STEP 15 – RIGHT ADRENAL GLAND

The adrenal gland is found on the palm slightly below where the thumb meets the hand in line with the webbing of the thumb and index finger. The right adrenal gland is very close to the kidney reflex point.

Support with your left hand and use the hook in and back-up technique to treat the adrenal reflex. It is usually a tender point.

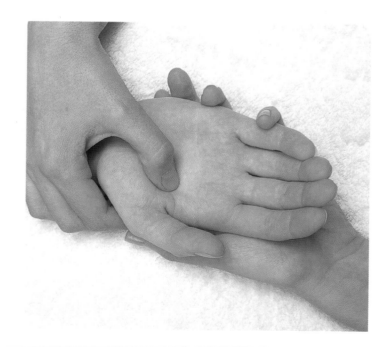

USES: Any condition where there is inflammation e.g. rheumatoid arthritis and irritable bowel syndrome, allergies. Also for stress, pain relief and lack of energy.

STEP 16 – RIGHT KIDNEY/URETER TUBE/BLADDER

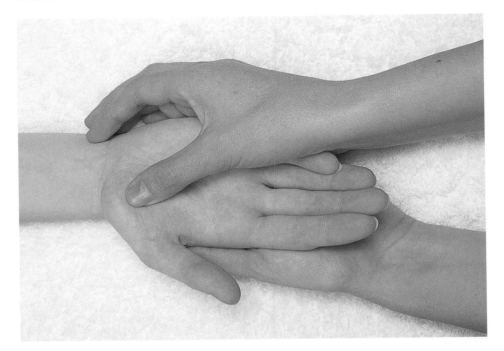

The bean-shaped kidney point is located on the palm of the hand in zones two and three on the waistline. It is just below the adrenal reflex so move your right thumb down and across to the right slightly and perform gentle pressure circles over the area.

Turn your thumb around and thumb walk down the hand towards zone 1 on the inside of the hand just above the wrist. This is the bladder area.

Perform pressure circles over this area.

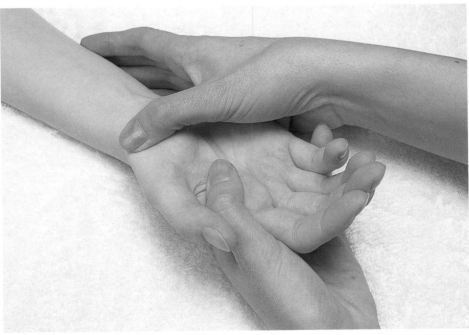

USES: Bladder infections, cystitis, fluid retention, bedwetting, incontinence.

NB: Never work upwards from the bladder towards the kidney or you could transform a mild bladder infection into a kidney infection which of course is much more serious.

STEP 17 – SMALL INTESTINES

The small intestine zone extends over zones one, two, three and four. Supporting the hand, palm uppermost, start just below the waist line and work from the inner aspect of the hand (i.e. thumb-side) across the palm of the hand to zone four.

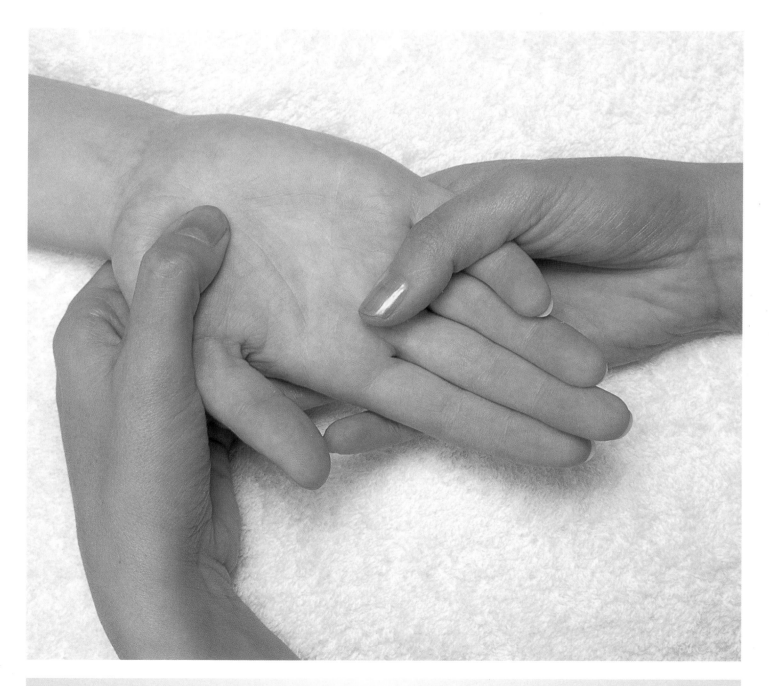

USES: All digestive problems including Crohn's disease and coeliac disease.

STEP 18 – ILEOCAECAL VALVE/ASCENDING AND TRANSVERSE COLON

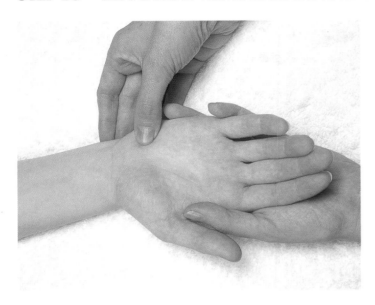

Support the hand palm uppermost with your left hand. The ileocaecal valve is found on the right hand only in zone 5 (little finger side) just above the wrist. Use your right thumb to perform the hook in and back-up technique or alternatively you may perform the rotation on the point technique.

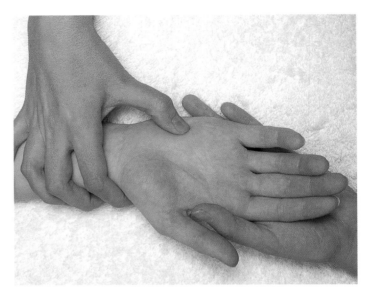

Thumb walk up zone 5 (ascending colon).

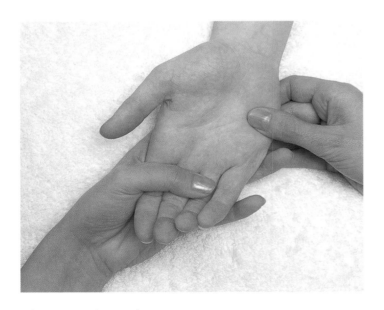

Then turn at the waistline.

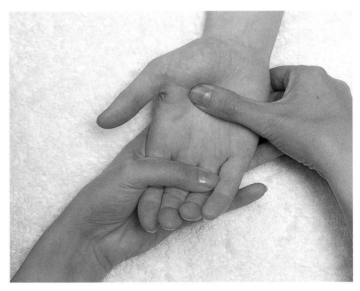

Walk across the hand finishing in the web of the thumb (across the first transverse part of the colon).

USES: Constipation, diarrhoea, diverticulitis, irritable bowel syndrome, ulcerative colitis, Crohn's disease.

STEP 19 – JOINTS: SHOULDER, ELBOW, HIP, KNEE, (OUTER EDGE OF THE HAND)

Holding with your left hand, thumb on top, fingers underneath, with the receiver's hand palm uppermost, use your right thumb to walk down the outer edge of the hand starting at the base of the little finger (shoulder joint).

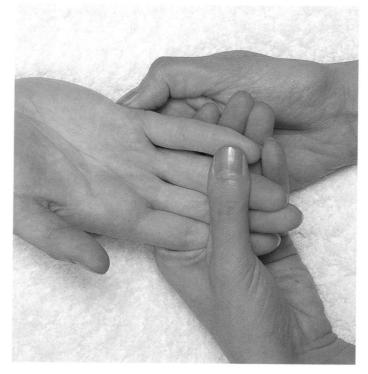

Continue walking down the edge of the hand with your thumb. To cover the reflex areas for the elbow, knee and hip joints.

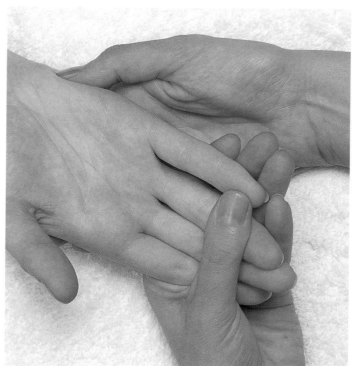

USES: Any problems with the joints including arthritis; frozen shoulder, tennis elbow, sprains, strains and sports injuries.

STEP 20 – RIGHT OVARY/TESTICLE

The reproductive areas are found around the wrist. The ovary is located on the outside on the wrist when it is palm down. Press your left thumb into the ovary reflex on the outer edge of the wrist and use the rotation on a point technique.

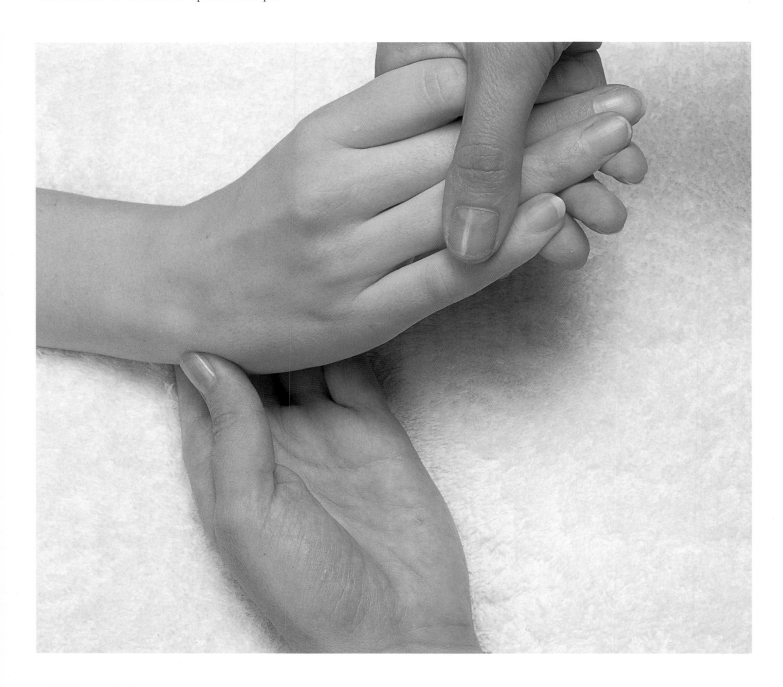

USES: Menstrual irregularities, ovarian cysts, infertility problems.

STEP 21 – UTERUS/PROSTATE

Locate the reflex on the inside of the wrist palm down with your right thumb. Use your left hand to perform the rotation around a point technique.

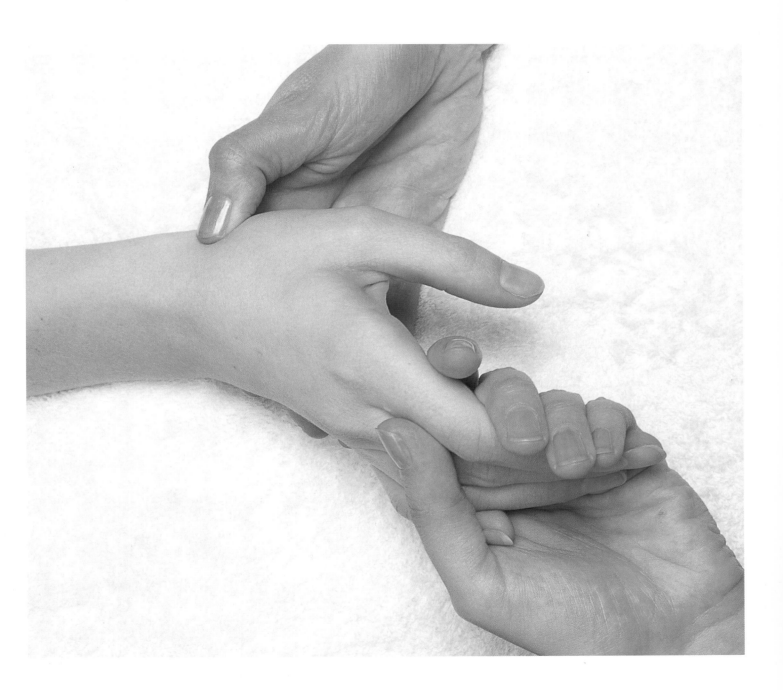

USES: Menstrual problems – painful, irregular, scanty or heavy menstruation, fertility problems, menopause, pre-menstrual syndrome, prostate problems.

STEP 22 – RIGHT FALLOPIAN TUBE/VAS DEFERENS/LYMPH NODES OF GROIN

The fallopian tube connects the ovary/uterus and the vas deferens
connects the testicle/prostate points together.

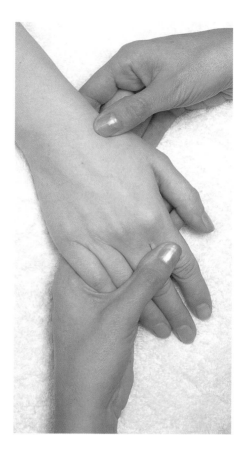

Thumb walk across the wrist on the back
of the hand.

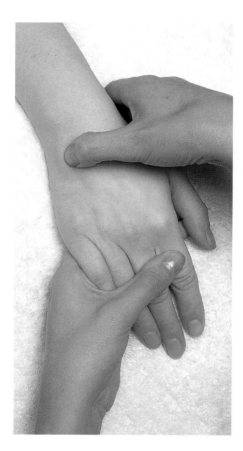

Continue thumb walking across the top
of the wrist.

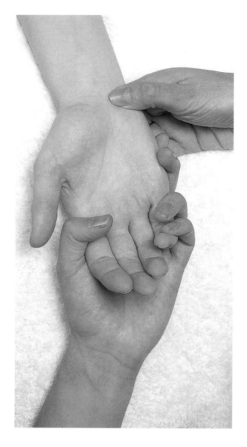

Then turn the hand over and thumb
walk across the wrist of the palm of the
hand to thoroughly work the pelvic
lymphatics.

USES: Problems with the male or female reproductive organs; to drain toxins; reduce fluid retention and
build up the body's defence system.

STEP 23 – COMPLETING THE RIGHT HAND

Perform gentle stroking movements on the top of the hand.

Then perform them on the palm of the hand. These will ensure that any toxins which have been released during the treatment are dispersed and will create a deep sense of relaxation.

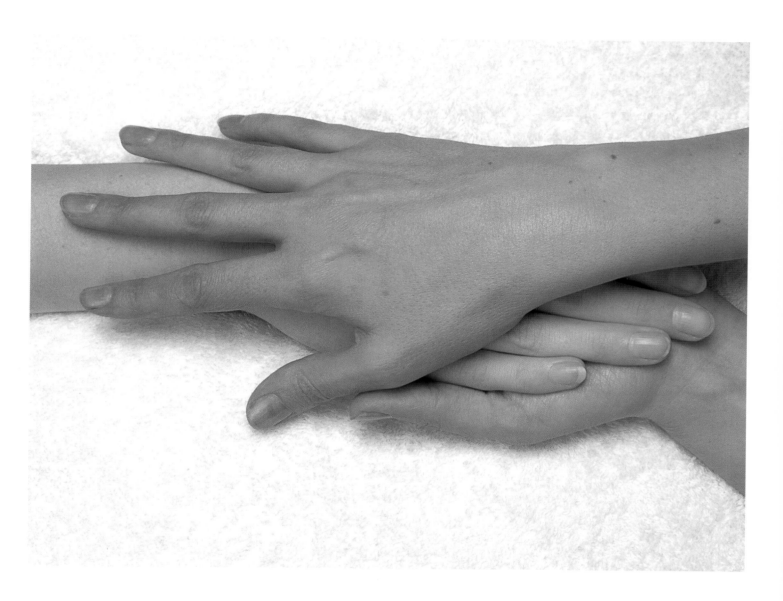

Left Hand

RELAXATION TECHNIQUES

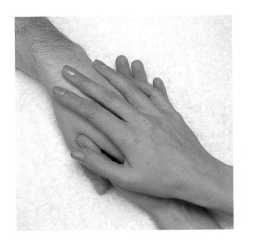

Greeting the hand

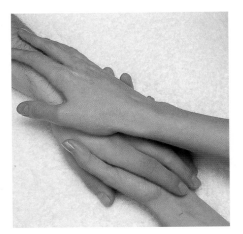

Stroking the hand and lower arm

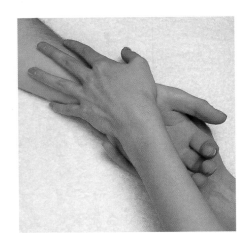

Stroking the hand – palm down

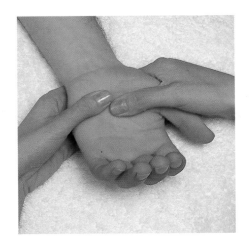

Opening the hand – palm up

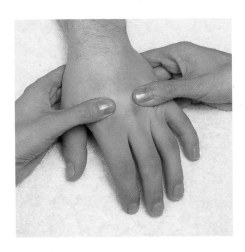

Opening the hand – palm down

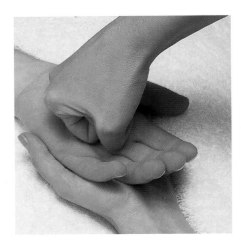

Knuckling the palm

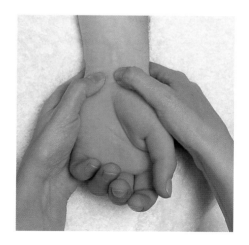

Loosening the wrist

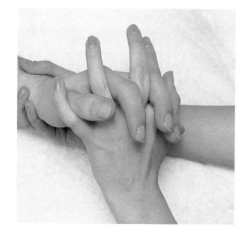

Moving the wrist backwards and forwards

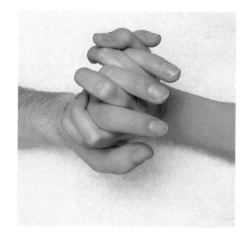

Rotating the wrist

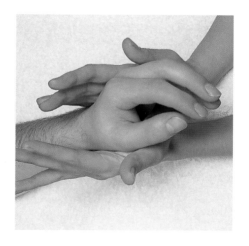

Wrist rolling

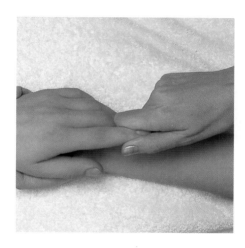

Streching the fingers and thumb

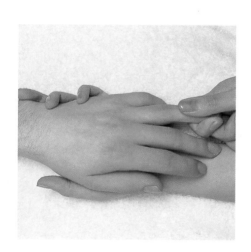

Loosening the fingers

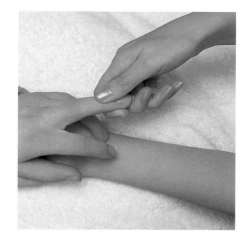

Moving the fingers and thumb

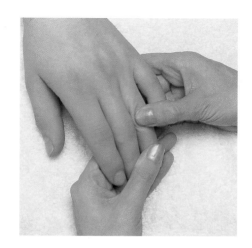

Circling the fingers and thumb

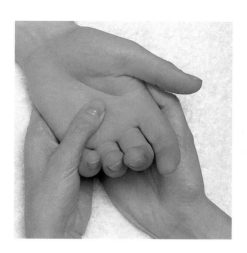

Solar plexus release

STEP 1 – HEAD AND BRAIN (SIDES OF THE THUMB)

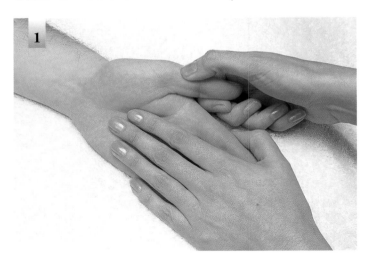

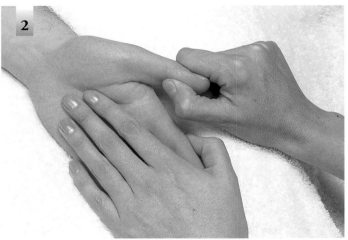

Start with the receiver's left hand, palm uppermost. Use your right thumb to walk from the very tip of the thumb down to the outside (1), down the back (2) and down the inside (3).

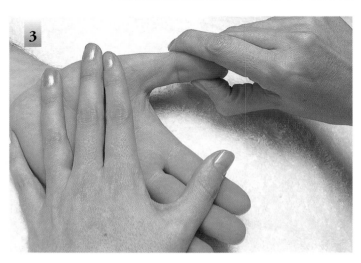

USES: Headaches and migraine. Any problems involving the brain, e.g. Parkinson's disease, Alzheimer's disease, stroke, lack of concentration, poor memory, cerebral palsy, multiple sclerosis and dyslexia.
It is also effective for lessening the after effects of an anaesthetic.

STEP 2 – PITUITARY GLAND (CENTRE OF THE BACK OF THE THUMB)

The pituitary gland is located approximately in the centre of the fleshy pad of the thumb – the thumb whorl. Support the thumb with the thumb and fingers of your holding hand. With your right thumb use the hook in and back-up technique on the pituitary reflex.

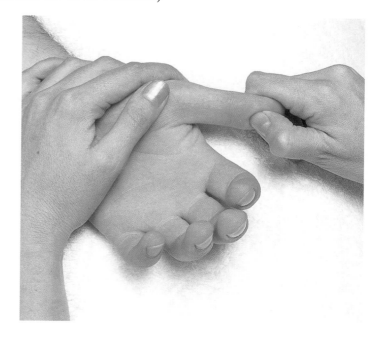

USES: All hormonal problems such as pre-menstrual syndrome and the menopause.
Any problems with the reproductive organs. Thyroid problems.

STEP 3 – FACE (FRONT OF THE THUMB)

Turn the hand over so that the palm is facing downwards and use your left thumb or index finger to work down the receiver's thumb from the tip to the base. Three or four rows should cover this area depending on the size of the thumb.

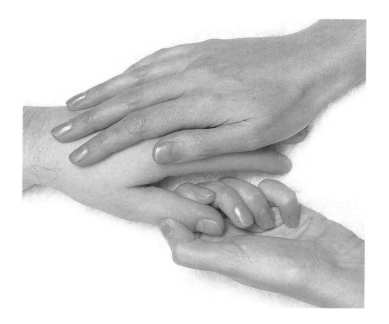

USES: Any problems involving the face including eye, nose, sinus, teeth, lips, gums, mouth and jaw problems.
This area is particularly effective for alleviating the excruciating pain of facial neuralgia and for Bell's palsy (facial paralysis).

STEP 4 – NECK ROTATION (BASE OF THE THUMB)

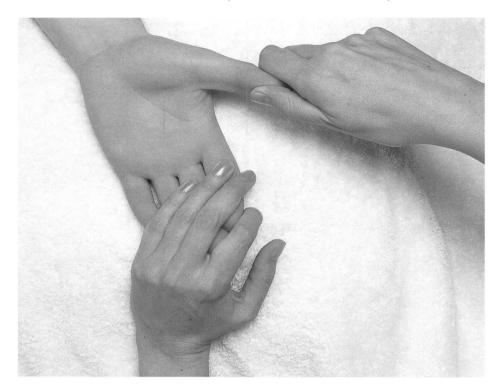

Turn the hand over, palm uppermost and grasp the thumb gently between your right thumb and index finger. Rotate it clockwise.

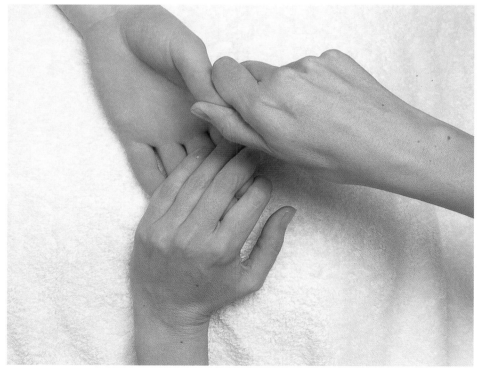

Repeat anti-clockwise. Rotating in both directions helps to counteract stiffness and increases movement in the neck.

USES: Neck pain, lack of mobility in the neck, whiplash injuries.

STEP – 5 NECK/THYROID (BACK AND FRONT OF THE BASE OF THE THUMB)

Stabilise the receiver's thumb between your left thumb and index finger. Use your right thumb to walk across the back of the base of the thumb.

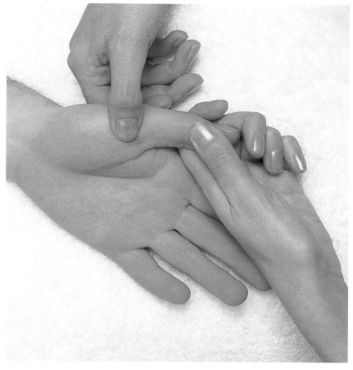

Now turn the hand over and using your left thumb, walk across the front of the base of the thumb.

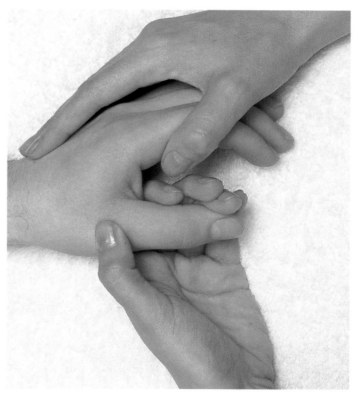

USES: All neck problems, disorders of the throat, tonsils and vocal cords, thyroid and parathyroid.

STEP 6 – SINUSES (BACK, SIDES AND TOP OF THE FINGERS)

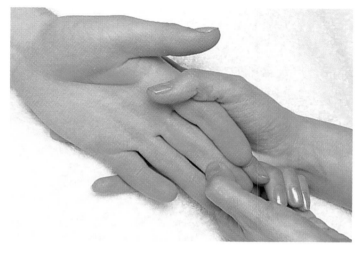

With the hand palm uppermost support the fingers with your right hand. Starting from the top of the little finger use your left thumb to walk down the finger. You will need about three to four rows of thumb walking to cover the back and sides of each finger thoroughly depending on size.

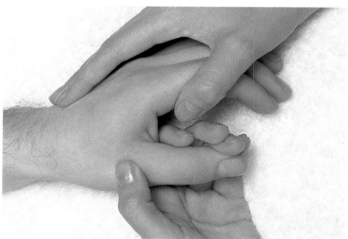

Repeat on each finger – you can if you wish use your right thumb to treat the index finger.

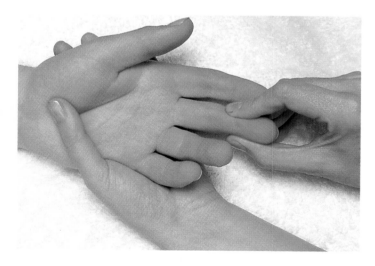

Alternatively when treating the sides of the fingers you may wish to use your thumb and index finger together.

USES: Sinus problems, hay fever, catarrh, allergies and colds.

STEP 7 – TEETH (DORSAL SIDE OF THE FINGERS)

Turn the hand over to work the dorsal side of the fingers. Starting at the tip of the index finger do three rows of finger walking down each finger.

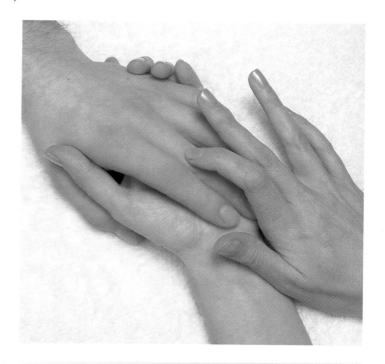

USES: Toothache; sensitive, infected or painful gums; abscesses.

STEP 8 – UPPER LYMPHATICS (WEBBING OF THE FINGERS)

Use your thumb and index finger to gently squeeze the webbing between the fingers. The webbing between the thumb and index finger is particularly effective.

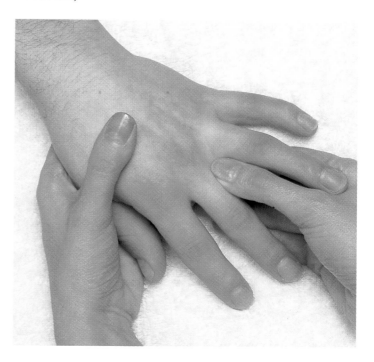

USES: To drain the head and neck; to fight off infection and boost the immune system.

STEP 9 – SPINE/SCIATIC LINE (INSIDE EDGE OF THE HAND/THE WRIST)

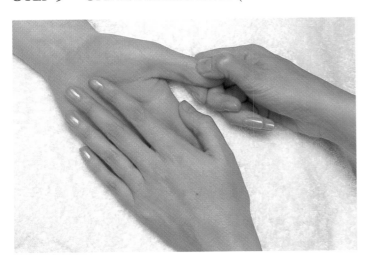

Sandwich the receiver's hand with your left hand on top of the palm. Starting at the first thumb joint walk your right thumb down the inside of the hand.

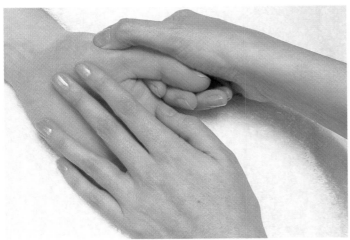

If you feel any 'gritty' areas as you work down then massage gently over them to thoroughly disperse any toxins.

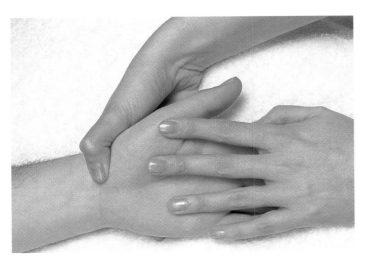

To treat the sciatic area continue walking across the wrist until you reach the other side of the hand.

USES: All back disorders including general aches and pains, degeneration of the spine, disc problems and sciatica.

STEP 10 – LEFT EYE AND EAR (BASE OF THE FINGERS)

Support the fingers between your left hand and use your right thumb to walk across the ridge at the base of the fingers working from the index finger across to zone 5.

Repeat the movement stopping between index and middle finger (eye point) and press and release several times.

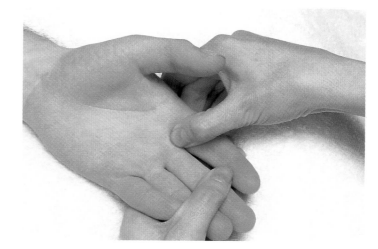

Walk a little further to between the third and fourth finger (eustachian tube) and press and release.

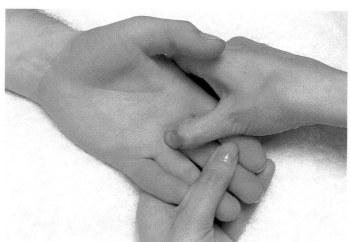

Continue to walk stopping between the fourth and fifth finger (ear point) and press and release.

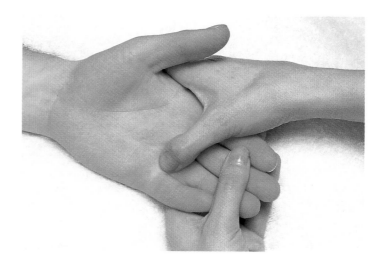

USES: All conditions involving the eyes including sore, tired or watery eyes, blocked tear ducts, glaucoma, cataracts and conjunctivitis. Ear problems such as ear infections, glue ear, tinnitus, vertigo and dizziness.

STEP 11 – LEFT LUNG/CHEST (PALM OF HAND)

The left lung occupies approximately the upper third of the hand. Support the receiver's hand, palm uppermost with your fingers of your left hand underneath and your left thumb on top pulling the fingers gently back. Use your right thumb to walk in horizontal strips across the hand working from the index finger to the little finger until you reach the diaphragm line. This should take approximately four rows.

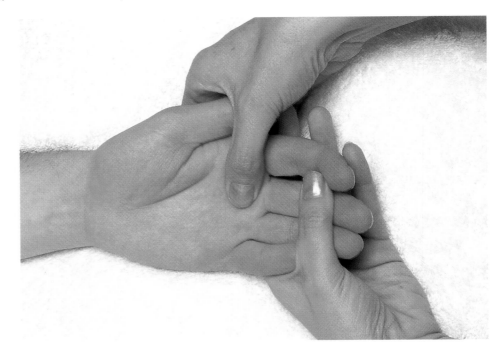

USES: All respiratory problems including chesty coughs, asthma, bronchitis, emphysema, pleurisy, hyperventilation and panic attacks.

STEP 12 – LEFT LUNG/BREAST/MAMMARY GLANDS (TOP OF HAND)

Turn the hand over. Supporting with your left hand and starting at the base of the fingers use your right index finger or index and middle finger to walk down the front of the upper third of the hand in vertical strips.

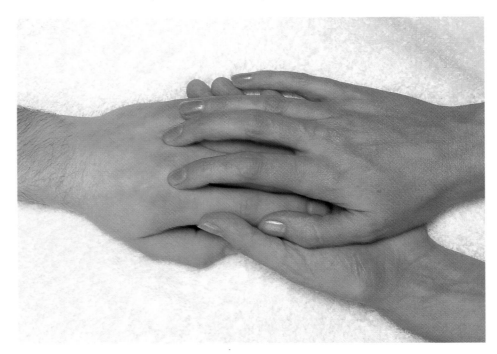

USES: All respiratory problems as described in Step 11. Also breast problems such as soreness due to pre-menstrual syndrome.

STEP 13 – HEART AREA – CARDIAC POINT (LEFT HAND ONLY)

The heart is treated on the left hand only. We have already treated the general heart area when working over the lungs and chest. The cardiac point is found on zone 4 slightly below the fourth finger. Locate the heart reflex and with your left thumb and perform several pressure circles over the area. Ensure that your pressure is very gentle and if there is any sensitivity do NOT increase the pressure.

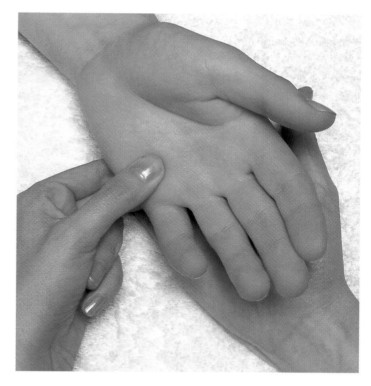

For a really gentle treatment on the heart, sandwich the receiver's hand palm uppermost between both your hands – one on the top, one underneath. Slowly and gently massage the palm of the receiver's hand in a circular direction with your left palm. At the same time massage the back of the receiver's hand with your right palm. This movement feels wonderful.

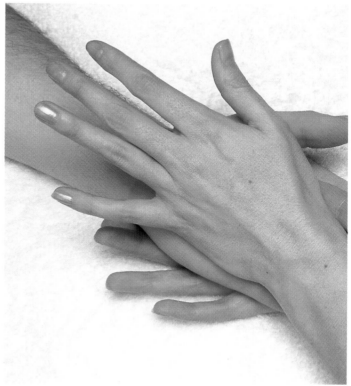

USES: All heart problems, palpitations, irregular heart beat, panic attacks.

STEP 14 – STOMACH/PANCREAS/DUODENUM

Supporting with your left hand, thumb on top, fingers underneath, use your right thumb to work across the palm of the hand as far as zone 3 from diaphragm line to waistline. Two to three horizontal rows should cover this area.

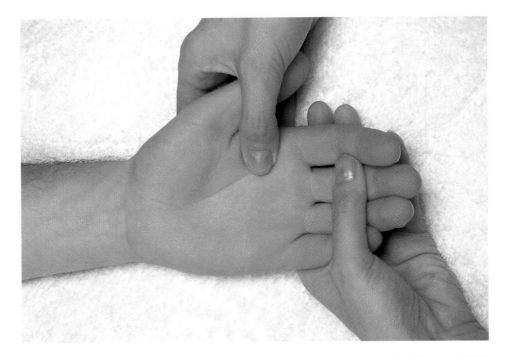

USES: Stomach problems including indigestion, hyperacidity, ulcers, general digestive disorders and diabetes.

STEP 15 – SPLEEN (LEFT HAND ONLY)

Support with your right hand, thumb on top, fingers underneath and with your left thumb work across the hand from zone five (little finger side) to zone four in horizontal rows.

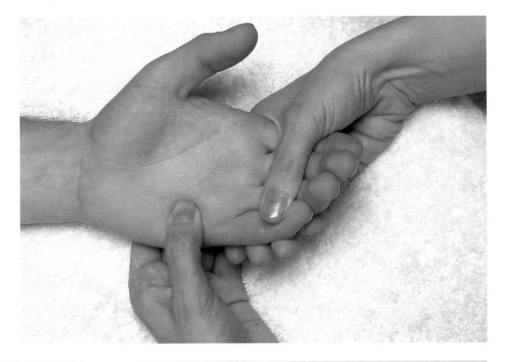

USES: To boost the immune system.

STEP 16 – LEFT ADRENAL GLAND

Locate the adrenal gland just below the webbing of the thumb and index finger. With your right thumb use the hook in and back-up technique on the adrenal reflex. If it is tender then do some gentle pressure circles over the area.

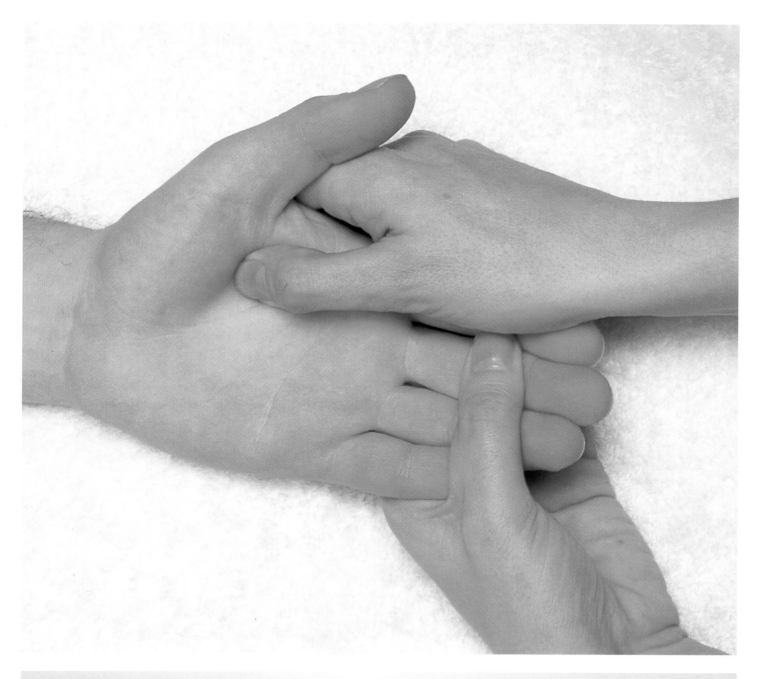

USES: Any condition where there is inflammation e.g. rheumatoid arthritis and irritable bowel syndrome, allergies. Also for stress, pain relief and lack of energy.

STEP 17 – LEFT KIDNEY /URETER TUBE/BLADDER

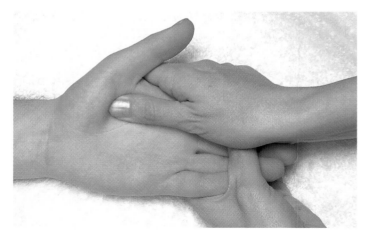

Move your right thumb down slightly and flatten the pad so that it is positioned on zones two and three. Perform gentle pressure circles over the area.

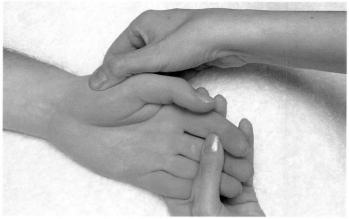

Turn your right thumb and walk down towards zone one on the inner aspect of the hand.

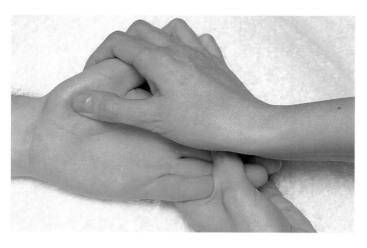

Perform gentle pressure circles over the bladder reflex. REMEMBER to always walk from kidney to bladder.

USES: Bladder infections, cystitis, fluid retention, bedwetting, incontinence.

NB: Never work upwards from the bladder towards the kidney or you could transform a mild bladder infection into a kidney infection which of course is much more serious.

STEP 18 – SMALL INTESTINES

Support the hand palm uppermost with your left hand. Using your right thumb work from zone one (thumb side) from just below the waistline as far as zone 4. This will take you about three or four horizontal rows.

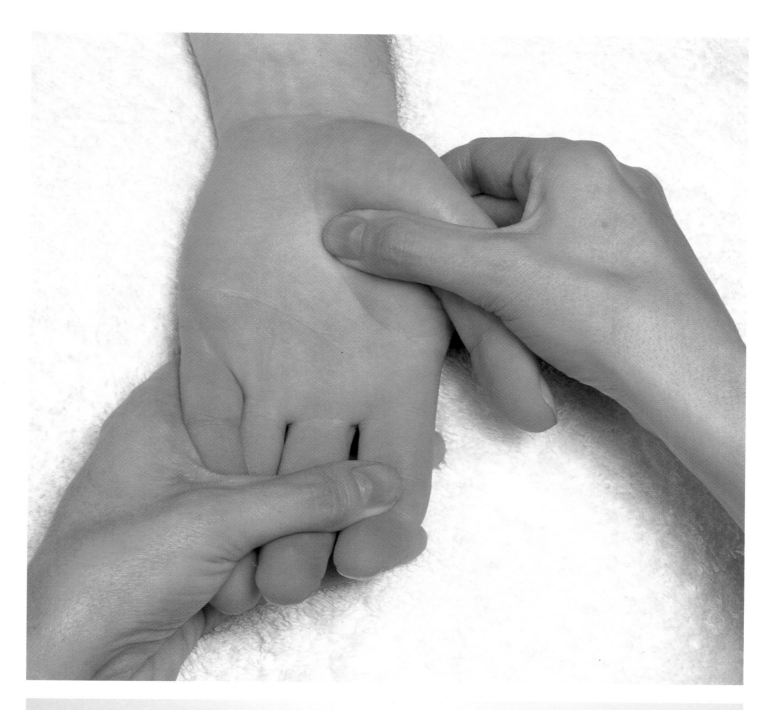

USES: All digestive problems including Crohn's disease and coeliac disease.

STEP 19 – TRANSVERSE/DESCENDING/SIGMOID COLON/RECTUM

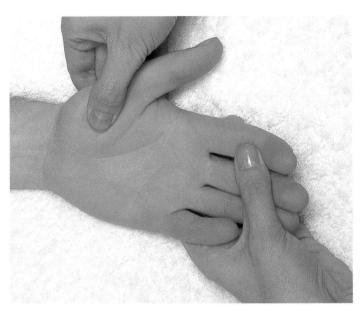

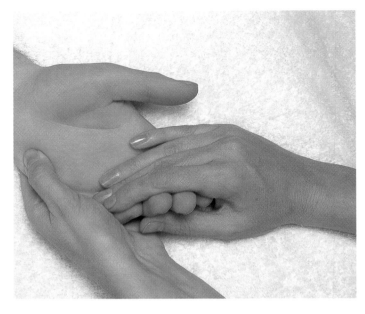

With the receiver's hand palm uppermost use your left hand as support, thumb on the top and fingers underneath. Use your right thumb to walk across the waistline (transverse colon) until you reach zone 5.

Change hands, and walk down the side of the hand (descending colon) with your left thumb.

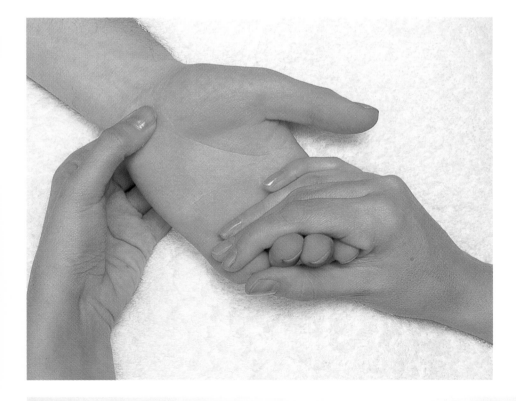

Before you reach the base of the palm turn your left thumb 90° and walk across the palm of the hand (sigmoid colon) to the inside of the wrist which is the rectum. Do some gentle pressure circles over this area.

USES: Constipation, diarrhoea, diverticulitis, irritable bowel syndrome, ulcerative colitis, Crohn's disease.

STEP 20 – JOINTS: SHOULDER, ELBOW, HIP, KNEE (OUTER EDGE OF THE HAND)

Hold the left hand, palm uppermost, with your right hand. Place your thumb on top of the palm, fingers underneath. Use your left thumb to walk down the outer edge of the hand starting at the base of the little finger (shoulder reflex).

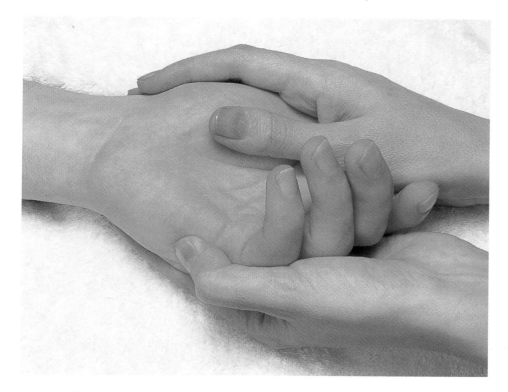

Continue working down the outer edge of the hand with your thumb until you reach the base of the palm.

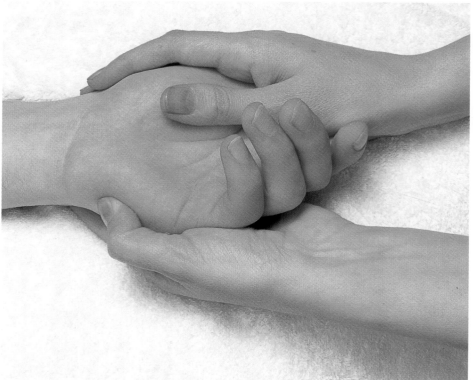

USES: Any problems with the joints including arthritis; frozen shoulder, tennis elbow, sprains, strains and sports injuries.

STEP 21 – LEFT OVARY/TESTICLE

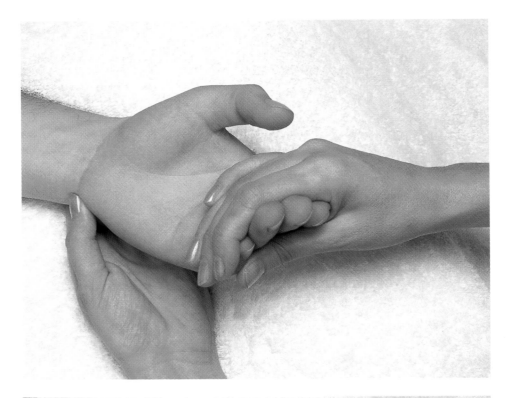

With the receiver's hand palm uppermost place your left thumb on the little finger side of the wrist into the ovary/testicle reflex point.

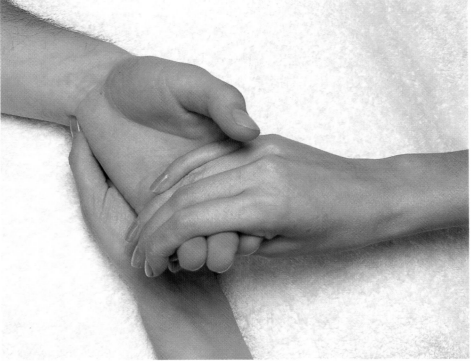

With your right hand rotate the receiver's hand around the point.

USES: Menstrual irregularities; ovarian cysts; infertility problems.

STEP 22 – UTERUS/PROSTATE

Locate the uterus/prostate reflex on the thumb side of the wrist.
Use your right thumb or index finger to perform the rotation on a
point technique.

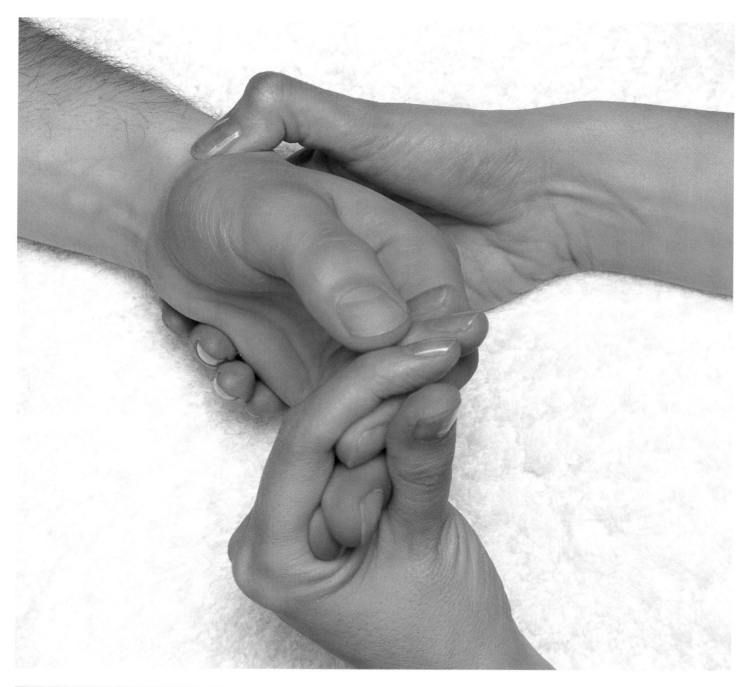

USES: Menstrual problems – painful, irregular, scanty or heavy menstruation, fertility problems, menopause,
pre-menstrual syndrome, prostate problems.

STEP 23 – LEFT FALLOPIAN TUBE/VAS DEFERENS/LYMPH NODES OF THE GROIN

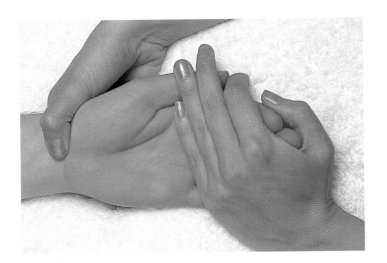

Thumb walk across the wrist. Begin on one side of the wrist, and walk right across.

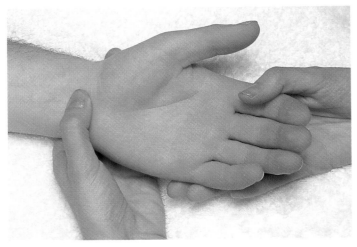

Now walk across the wrist beginning at the other side.

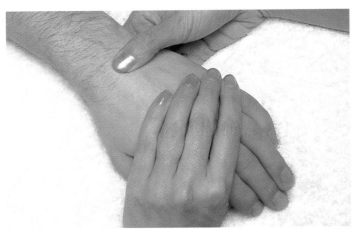

Now turn the hand over and again thumb walk across the wrist in both directions.

USES: Problems with the male or female reproductive organs, to drain toxins, reduce fluid retention and build up the body's defence system.

STEP 24 – COMPLETING THE LEFT HAND

Stroke the left hand gently using both your hands to disperse any toxins. Well done —the sequence is now complete.

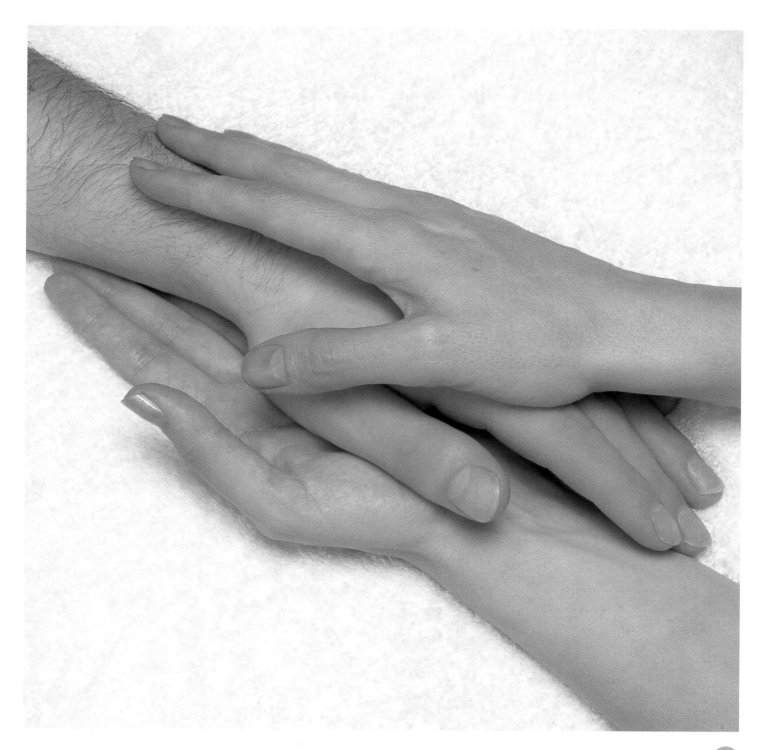

CLOSING MOVEMENTS

1. Return to any reflex areas that were sensitive during the treatment.

2. Carry out any of your favourite relaxation techniques. You may decide to use an oil or cream to moistutise the hands. There are several recipes in the self treatment section of this book.

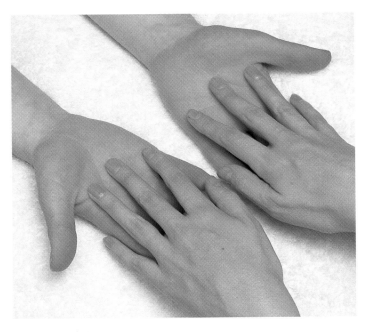

3. Run your fingertips gently down both of the hands.

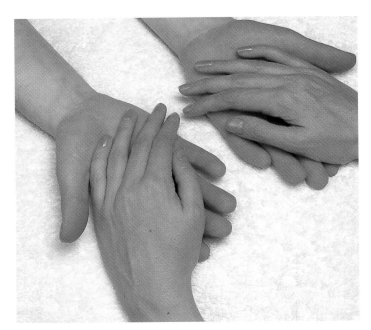

4. Clasp both hands in your hands and hold for a few seconds.

5. Cover up the hands and allow the receiver to relax for a few minutes.

6. On your return offer them a large glass of water and encourage them to drink 6–8 glasses over the next 24 hours to flush away the toxins.

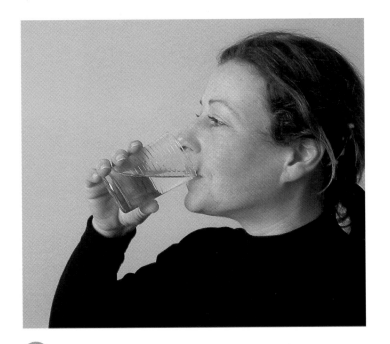

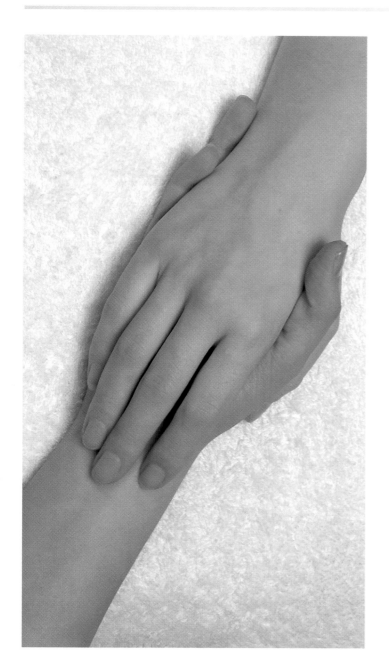

Hand reflexology is the ideal therapy for self-treatment. The hands are an excellent place to work on yourself as you can easily reach all the reflex areas.

Reflexology areas can be massaged at any time of the day and in any place. No one will even know that you are treating yourself. You can do it travelling on the bus or train to work, sitting in your office in your tea or lunch break or whilst you are watching television in the evening. You can even carry out hand reflexology standing up. Why not try it next time you are standing in a long queue in the supermarket or waiting for transportation – especially if delayed at airports.

Whenever you get a moment to relax why not work on your hands not only as a means of relaxation but also as a way of maintaining good health. Never be worried that you will harm yourself. Reflexology is perfectly safe provided it is used correctly. The main points to remember are do NOT work too deeply on a reflex area and do NOT work for too long on a particular area otherwise areas can become over-stimulated and a side-effect such as diarrhoea could be experienced.

BASIC HAND REFLEXOLOGY ROUTINE

Try the following simple routine at least once a week. It should take you about 15 minutes.

Positions For Working

You need to be seated comfortably for your self-reflexology session perhaps in your favourite chair or even on the floor with a pillow or cushion on your lap.

Alternatively you can sit with your hand resting on a pillow or cushion on top of a table. The table should be the right height that you don't have to reach up and you should make sure that you are fairly close to it so that you do not have to lean too far forward.

Rest your hand gently on the cushion, check your posture relaxing your shoulders and wrists and off you go!

LEFT HAND

STEP 1 – HEAD/BRAIN/FACE (THUMB)

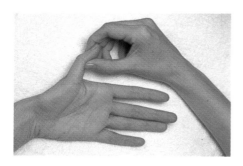

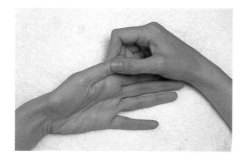

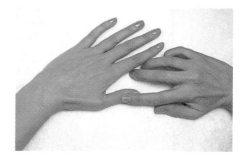

With your right thumb walk down the back of your left thumb starting at the very tip.

Then thumb walk down the sides of your thumb.

Now use your index finger to walk down the front of the thumb (face).

STEP 2 – PITUITARY GLAND (CENTRE OF THUMB)

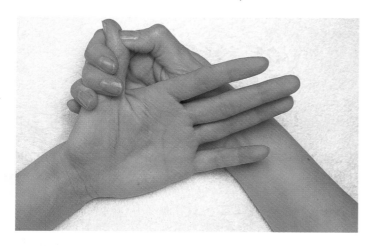

Locate the pituitary gland in the centre of the fleshy pad of the thumb. Use the hook in and back-up technique.

STEP 3 – NECK/THYROID (BASE OF THE THUMB)

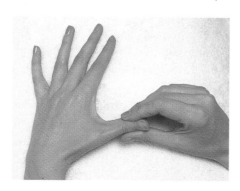

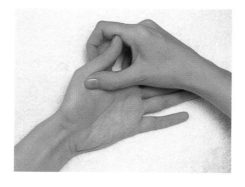

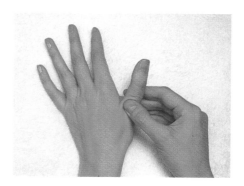

Grasp the left thumb between your right thumb and index finger and rotate it slowly and gently to loosen your neck.

Use your right thumb to walk across the base of the back of the thumb.

Then walk down the front of the thumb. This will treat the neck, thyroid, parathyroid and any throat disorders.

STEP 4 – SINUSES (BACK, SIDES AND TOP OF THE FINGERS)
TEETH (FRONT OF THE FINGERS)

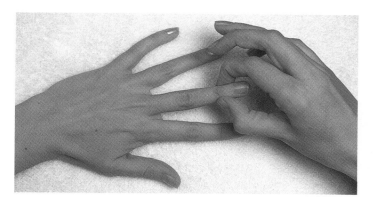

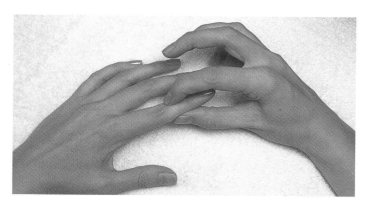

Use your thumb and index finger working together to walk down the sides of each finger.

Now use your right thumb and index finger to walk down the front and back of each finger.

STEP 5 – UPPER LYMPHATICS (WEBS OF THE FINGERS)

Use your thumb and index finger to gently squeeze between each of the fingers.

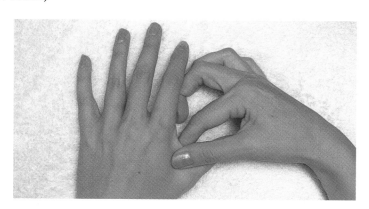

STEP 6 – SPINE (INSIDE EDGE (THUMB SIDE) OF THE HAND)

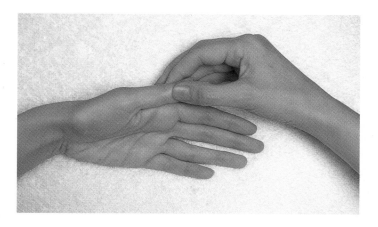

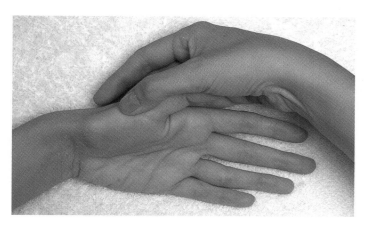

Rest your hand palm uppermost and walk your right thumb down the inside of your hand. Begin at the tip of the thumb (neck/cervical area).

Continue walking down to the wrist (lumbar area).

STEP 7 – EYES AND EARS (BASE OF THE FINGERS)

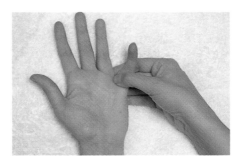

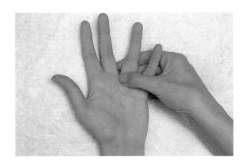

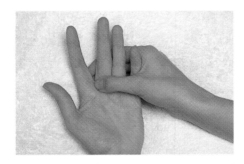

Walk across the ridge at the base of the fingers working from zone 5. Press into the ear point between fingers 4 and 5.

Then press on the eustachian tube point, situated between fingers 3 and 4.

Finally press the eye point between the index and middle finger. Use pressure circles to disperse any crystals.

STEP 8 – LEFT LUNG/CHEST (UPPER THIRD OF THE PALM OF THE HAND)

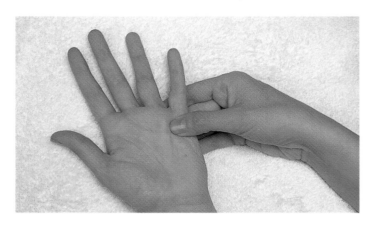

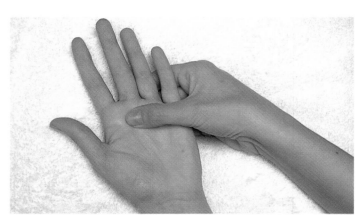

Thumb walk from zone 5 (little finger side) across the upper third of the hand in horizontal rows until you reach the diaphragm line.

STEP 9 – LEFT LUNG/BREAST/MAMMARY GLANDS

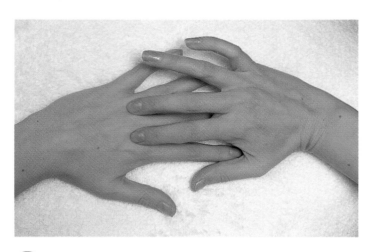

Turn the hand over palm facing down and use your index and middle finger (you can also use your index finger only) to walk down the hand, starting at the base of the fingers.

STEP 10 – STOMACH/PANCREAS/DUODENUM/SPLEEN

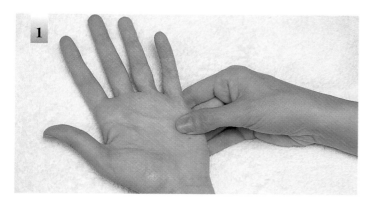

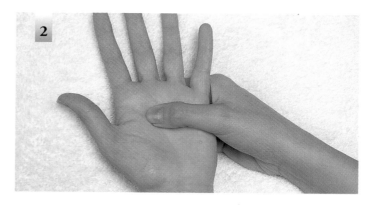

Turn the hand palm uppermost and thumb walk in horizontal rows across the hand from zone 5 (little finger side) towards the

thumb. You are treating the spleen as you work over zones 4-5 (1), the stomach, pancreas and duodenum in zones 1-3 (2).

STEP 11 – LEFT ADRENAL GLAND/KIDNEY/URETER TUBE/BLADDER

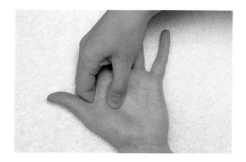

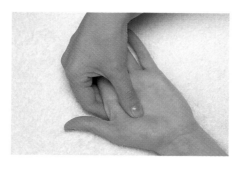

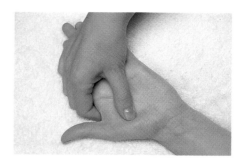

Use the hook in and back-up technique with your right thumb on the adrenal gland reflex which is found just below the webbing of the thumb and index finger.

Flatten the thumb to locate the kidney reflex and perform gentle pressure circles over the area.

Walk diagonally down towards the inside of the hand. Massage the bladder area gently.

STEP 12 – SMALL INTESTINES

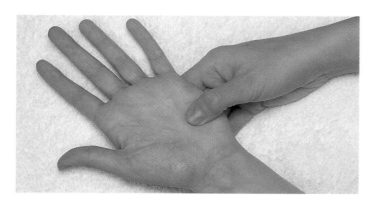

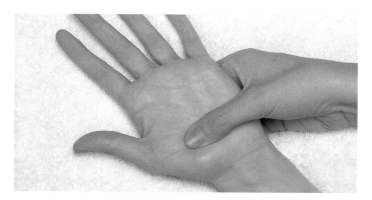

Thumb walk across the lower third of the palm of the hand in horizontal rows. Remember to stop and work gently into any sensitive areas.

STEP 13 – TRANSVERSE/DESCENDING/SIGMOID COLON/RECTUM

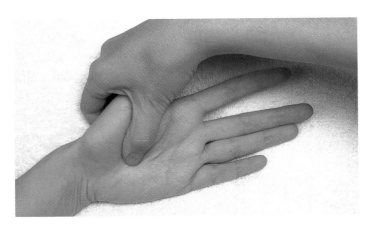

Commencing just below the thumb walk across the palm of the hand (transverse colon).

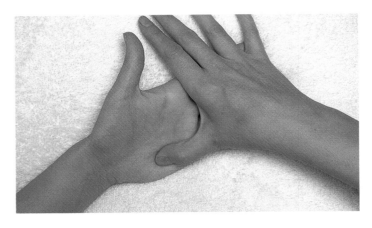

Turn at zone 5 and walk down the hand (descending colon).

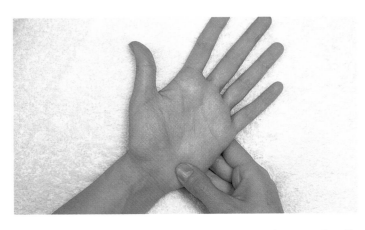

Just before you reach the wrist, turn the thumb 90° and walk across to zone 1 (rectum).

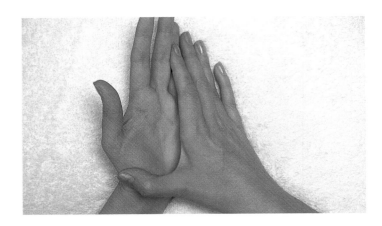

Do a few pressure circles over the rectum.

STEP 14 – JOINTS AND SCIATIC LINE (OUTER EDGE OF HAND)

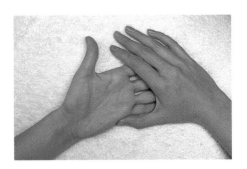

With palm uppermost, walk down the outer edge of the hand starting at the base of the little finger (shoulder reflex).

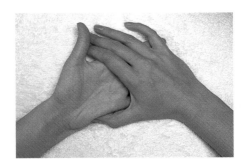

Continue thumb walking down this outer edge.

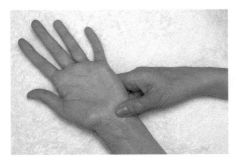

When you reach the wrist, continue to walk across the wrist until you reach the other side of the hand (sciatic line).

STEP 15 – LEFT OVARY/TESTICLE/UTERUS/PROSTATE

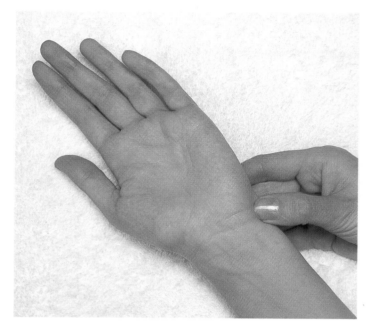

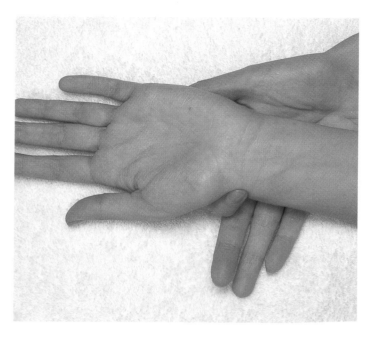

With the palm uppermost use your right thumb to perform pressure circles on the ovary/testicle reflex on the outside of the wrist.

Then use your index finger to treat the uterus/prostate on the inside of the wrist.

STEP 16 – LEFT FALLOPIAN TUBE/VAS DEFERENS/LYMPH NODES OF THE GROIN

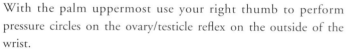

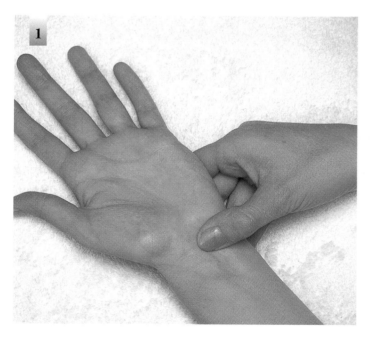

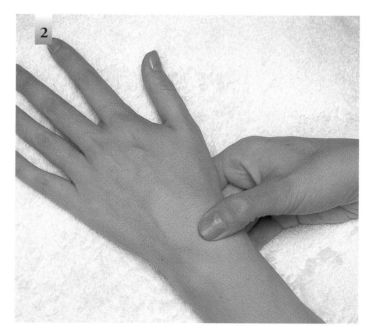

Use your right thumb or index finger to walk all the way around your left wrist – front (1) and back (2).

Right Hand

STEP – 1 Head/brain/face (Thumb)

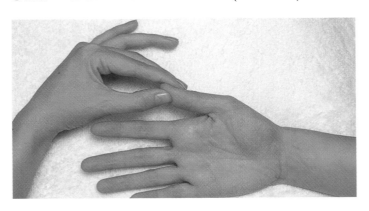

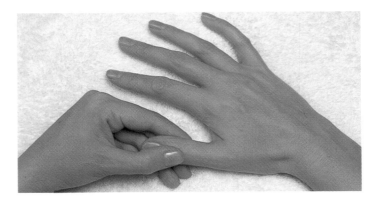

With the palm uppermost use your left thumb to walk down the back and sides of your right thumb.

Turn the hand over and use your thumb or index finger to walk down the front of the thumb (face).

STEP 2 – Pituitary gland (Centre of thumb)

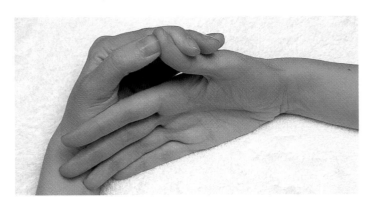

Find the pituitary gland approximately in the centre of the thumb. Use your left thumb to hook in and back-up on the reflex point.

STEP 3 – Neck/thyroid (Base of the thumb)

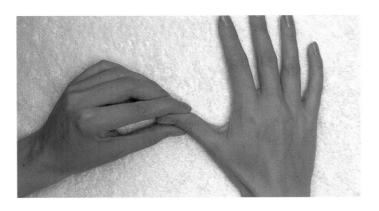

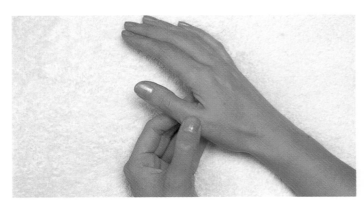

Hold your right thumb between your left thumb and forefinger and circle it clockwise and anti-clockwise.

With your right palm facing downwards walk across the front of the base of the thumb with your left thumb whilst you walk across the bottom with your index finger.

STEP 4 – SINUSES (BACK, SIDES AND TOP OF THE FINGERS) TEETH (FRONT OF THE FINGERS)

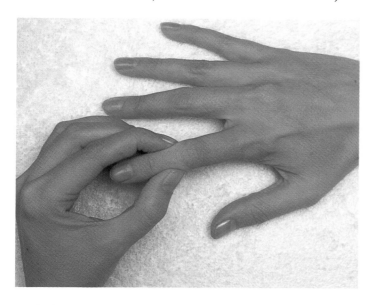

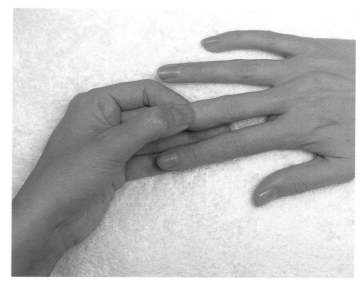

With the palm facing downwards use your left thumb and index finger to walk down the sides of each finger.

Now use your thumb and index finger to walk down the front and back of each finger with your thumb working on top and your index finger underneath.

STEP 5 – UPPER LYMPHATICS (WEBS OF THE FINGER)

Gently squeeze the webbing between the fingers with your left thumb and index finger.

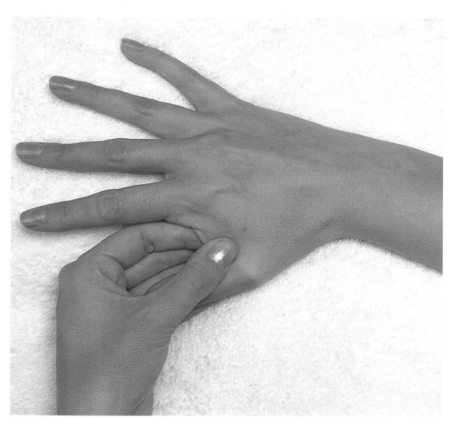

STEP 6 – SPINE (INNER EDGE OF THE HAND)

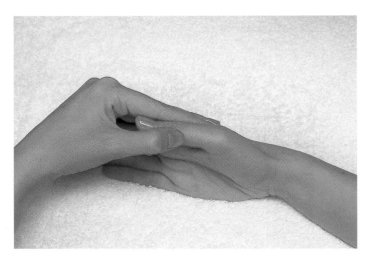

With your palm uppermost caterpillar walk your thumb down the inner edge of the hand (thumb side). Gently massage any gritty or tender areas. Continue to walk across the wrist to treat the sciatic area.

STEP 7 – EYES AND EARS (BASE OF THE FINGERS)

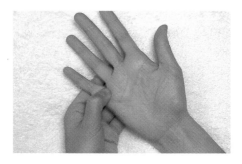

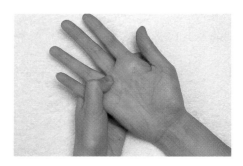

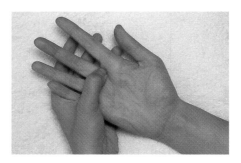

Support your right hand with your left hand, thumb on top, fingers underneath. Using your left thumb walk across the ridge at the base of the fingers. Stop between fingers 4 and 5 to press into the ear point.

Press between fingers 3 and 4 (eustachian tube point).

Now press between the index and middle finger (eye point).

STEP 8 – RIGHT LUNG/CHEST (UPPER THIRD OF THE PALM OF THE HAND)

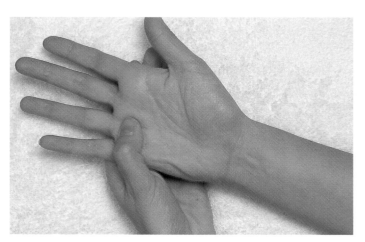

Thumb walk from zone 5 (little finger side) in horizontal strips across the hand as far as the diaphragm line.

STEP 9 – RIGHT LUNG/BREAST/MAMMARY GLANDS

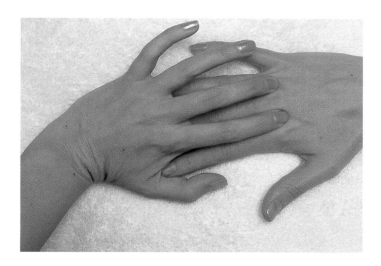

Turn the hand over and use your index and middle fingers (or your index finger alone) to walk down the hand in vertical strips starting from the base of the fingers.

STEP 10 – LIVER/GALLBLADDER (RIGHT HAND ONLY)

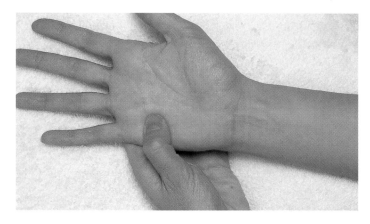

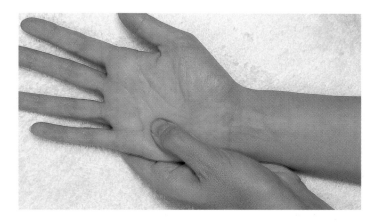

Supporting your hand palm uppermost, thumb on top and fingers underneath, walk from zone 5 (little finger side) to zone 3 from the diaphragm line to the waistline to cover the liver reflex.

To treat the gallbladder search the liver area under the region of the fourth finger and hook in and back-up.

STEP 11 – STOMACH/PANCREAS/DUODENUM

Now walk from zone 3 to zone 1 to treat the remaining area in horizontal rows.

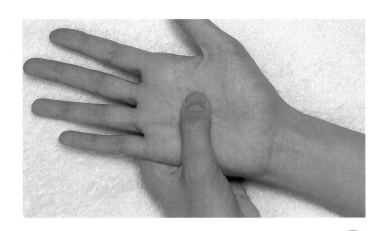

STEP 12 – RIGHT ADRENAL GLAND/KIDNEY/URETER TUBE/BLADDER

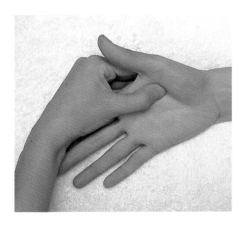 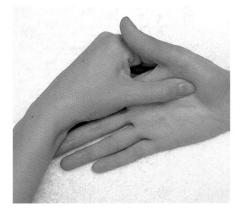 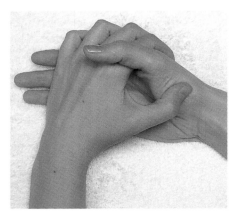

Hook in and back-up on the adrenal reflex which is located slightly below the webbing of the thumb and index finger. It is usually quite sensitive.

Flatten your thumb over the kidney area and perform gentle pressure circles.

Walk diagonally down towards zone 1 on the inner aspect of the hand. Gently massage the bladder area.

STEP 13 – SMALL INTESTINES

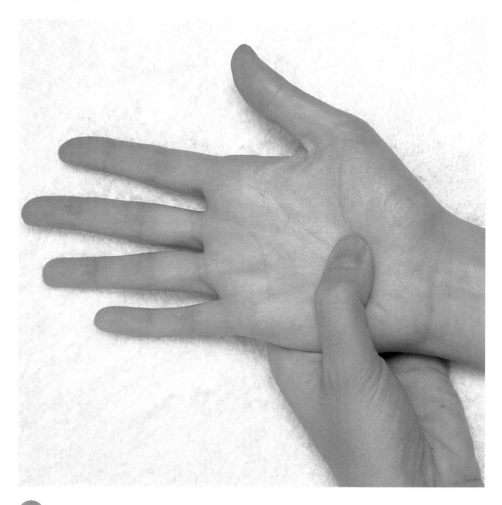

Supporting the hand palm uppermost work across the lower third of the palm of the hand from the outer aspect of the hand (little finger side) towards zone one.

STEP 14 – ILEOCAECAL VALVE/ASCENDING/TRANSVERSE COLON

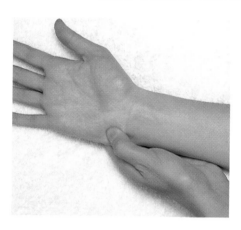 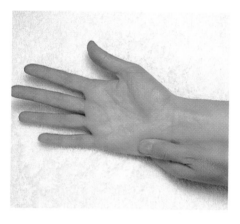 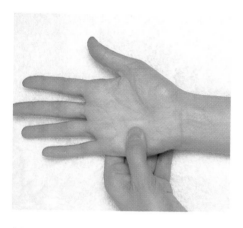

Locate the ileocaecal valve in zone 5 just above the wrist and hook in and back-up.

Thumb walk up zone 5 (ascending colon).

Turn at the waistline and walk across the transverse colon finishing at the base of the thumb.

STEP 15 – JOINTS AND SCIATIC LINE (OUTER EDGE OF HAND)

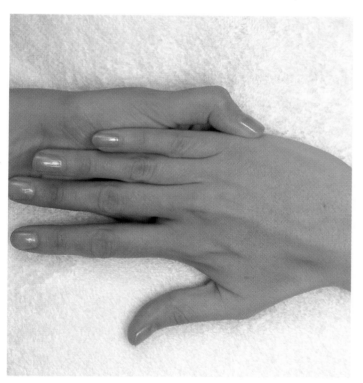 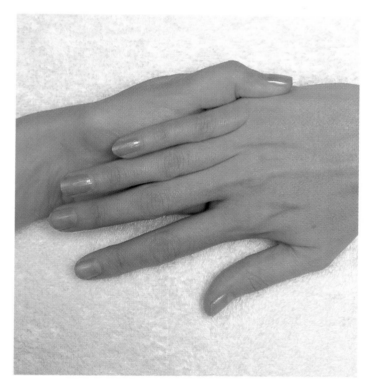

Turn your right hand round, palm down, with your fingertips towards you on the palm of your left hand. Use your left thumb to walk down the outer edge of the hand begining at the base of the little finger.

Continue thumb walking down the outside edge towards the wrist.

STEP 16 – RIGHT OVARY/TESTICLE/UTERUS/PROSTATE

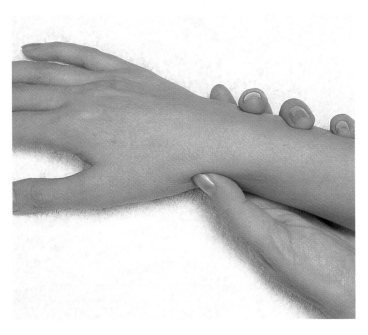

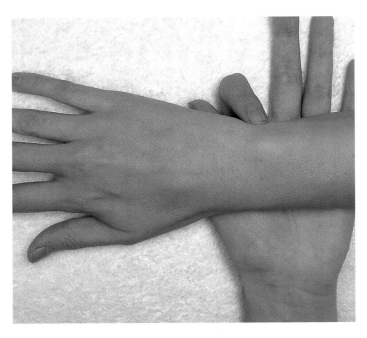

With your right palm down use your left thumb to locate and massage the uterus/prostate reflex on the inside of the wrist.

Use your left index finger to treat the ovary/testicle reflex on the outside (little finger side) of the wrist.

STEP 17 – RIGHT FALLOPIAN TUBE/VAS DEFERENS/LYMPH NODES OF THE GROIN

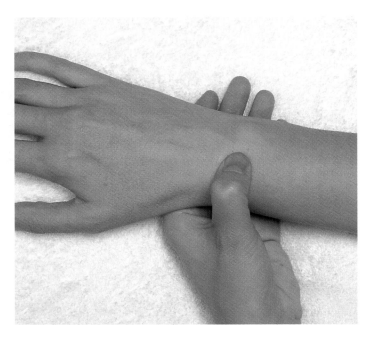

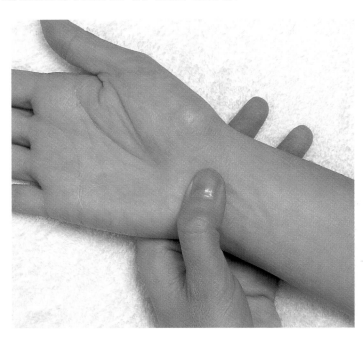

Now work right the way round the wrist using your left thumb or index finger.

Continue thumb walking over the whole wrist–both sides.

HAND HEALTH

Well done – you have carried out a complete hand reflexology treatment on yourself. You should feel wonderfully relaxed and revitalised. It is so important to take care of your hands – you owe it to yourself to look after your health. Many people devote a lot of time to their faces but forget about their hands. But the hands give the game away – our hands reflect our age as the skin becomes loose and wrinkled and age spots appear! Below are some tips to keep your hands looking their best.

HAND CARE TIPS

Massage pure creams into your hands regularly to keep them soft and moisturised. Remember they are permanently on display! Why not add essential oils to your hand creams to enhance your skin care. Here are some useful recipes to experiment with:

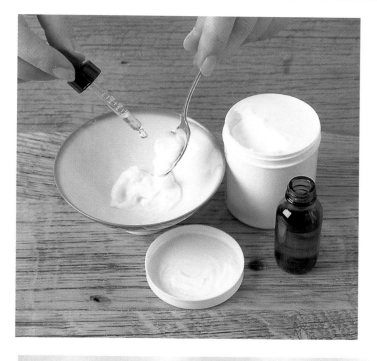

DRY/CRACKED/CHAPPED HANDS

To 30g cream add:
Three drops benzoin
Two drops myrrh
Two drops patchouli

or

To 30g cream add:
Four drops lavender
Three drops sandalwood

ITCHY/SENSITIVE/IRRITATED HANDS

To 30g cream add:
Three drops chamomile (Roman or German)
Four drops lavender

Everyday Hand Cream

To 30g cream add:
Three drops geranium
Four drops lavender

Warts – these are very common on the fingers and hands and although they will eventually go away on their own, essential oils can speed up their departure. With a cotton bud apply essential oils of LEMON or TEA TREE to the warts. Take care not to get too much essential oil on the surrounding area. Apply at least twice a day.

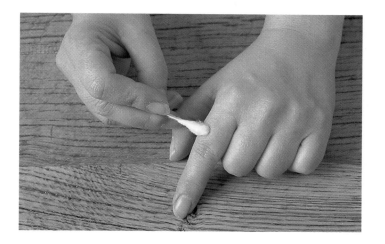

Exercise your hands regularly to keep them supple, healthy and to reduce tension. Below are some useful exercises that can help.

1. Hold a small ball in your hand and squeeze and relax your fingers around the ball repeatedly. Repeat with your other hand. This exercise will increase flexibility and strength.

2. Shake your hands out from the wrists as loosely and rapidly as possible to reduce tension (mental and physical).

3. Relax your fingers and circle both wrists clockwise and anti-clockwise. This helps to keep the wrists flexible and reduces puffiness.

4. Place the palms of your hands together in a prayer position. Rub your hands together rapidly in a backwards and forwards motion. Notice the heat produced by this movement and how invigorated you feel!

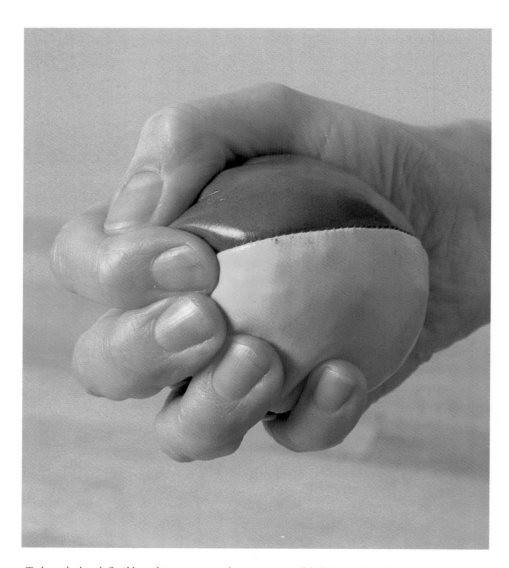

To keep the hands flexible and increase strength, squeeze a small ball in your hand.

hand reflexology for
Common Ailments

In the course of a hand reflexology treatment, disorders may show up as tender areas.

IMPORTANT:
All medical conditions should be checked by a fully qualified medical doctor.

It is always much more beneficial to carry out a complete reflexology treatment on both hands and then give additional attention to the tender reflex points. However, if time is short then it will be beneficial to concentrate on the areas indicated.

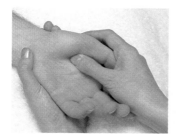

Adrenals

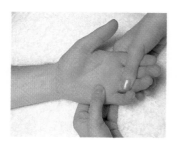

Diaphragm

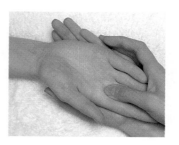

Eyes

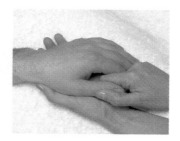

Face

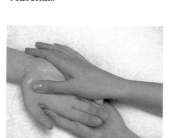

Kidneys

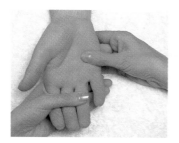

Ears

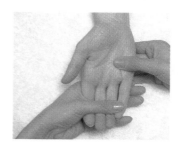

Liver

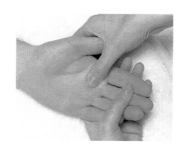

Lung/Chest Area

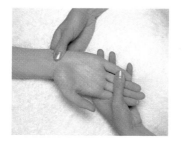

Lymphatics (Grain)

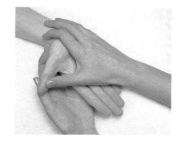

Pituitary gland

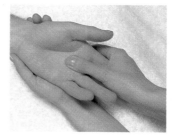

Solar Plexus

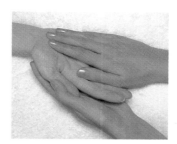

Spine

BLADDER PROBLEMS

CYSTITIS

This is an inflammation of the inner lining of the bladder usually caused by an infection entering the bladder via the urethral opening. The bacteria can come from the vagina or from the intestines via the anus. The symptoms include a frequent desire to urinate, often with a burning sensation. The urine may be stained with blood and there may be a fever.

General advice
- Drink lots of fluid to flush out the bladder. Cranberry juice is particularly helpful.

Reflexology Treatment

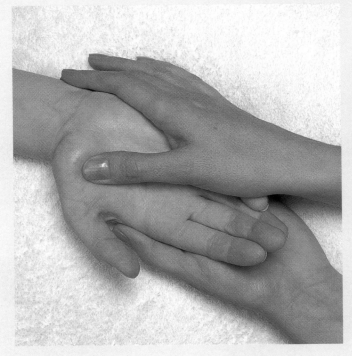

Kidney

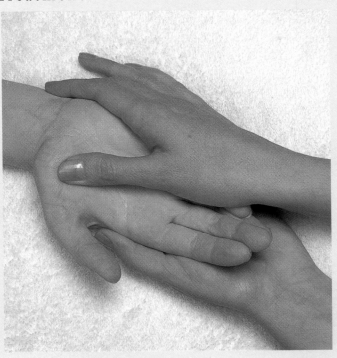

Working down the ureter tube towards the bladder

- Bladder
- Kidneys
- Ureter tubes
- Lymphatics

NB – always work from the kidney to the bladder and NEVER from the bladder to the kidney to avoid the risk of transferring a bladder infection into a kidney infection, which is far more serious.

DIGESTIVE PROBLEMS

CONSTIPATION

Constipation is commonly caused by a diet low in fibre; inadequate intake of water; lack of exercise; anxiety and certain medications such as excessive laxatives which make the bowel lazy; pain killers and antibiotics. It is characterised by the infrequent passage of hard stools usually with some discomfort.

General advice
- Eat a healthy, high-fibre diet to increase the frequency and quantity of bowel movements
- Avoid stress
- Do not ignore the urge to move your bowels
- Avoid laxatives

Reflexology Treatment

- Ileocaecal valve – which controls movement between the small and large intestines
- Small intestines
- Large intestines
- Adrenal glands
- Solar plexus – to reduce tension

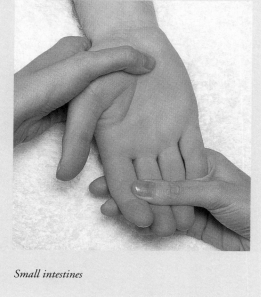

Small intestines

INDIGESTION /HEARTBURN

This is a very common problem giving symptoms of a taste of acid in the mouth and pain in the chest sometimes with nausea. It is caused by eating the wrong foods such as cakes and biscuits; fatty foods; hot and spicy foods; rich or dairy foods. Rushing or not chewing food properly and stress will also exacerbate acidity.

General advice
- Avoid stress and learn to relax
- Reduce acid – forming foods
- Chew food slowly in pleasant surroundings

Reflexology Treatment

- Stomach/pancreas/ duodenum
- Solar plexus – to reduce stress
- Adrenal glands – to reduce inflammation
- Liver/gallbladder – where there is nausea

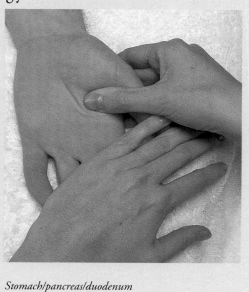

Stomach/pancreas/duodenum

FEMALE PROBLEMS

Ailments falling into this category include pre-menstrual syndrome (PMS); painful, absent or scanty periods; menopause; fibroids in the uterus; ovarian cysts and infertility problems.

General advice
- Eat a healthy diet
- Reduce sugar and caffeine, which aggravate mood swings
- Take vitamin B complex
- Take regular, gentle exercise such as yoga and Tai Chi
- If menopausal eat foods rich in calcium – e.g. fish where the bones are eaten, such as sardines, nuts and seeds.

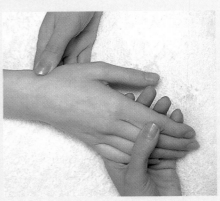

Reflexology Treatment

Ovaries

- Ovaries (illustrated using index finger)
- Uterus (illustrated using thumb)
- Fallopian tubes
- Kidneys – where there is excessive fluid

Uterus

- Breasts – where there is soreness
- Pituitary gland – to balance hormones
- Solar plexus – to relax
- Spine – for back pain

HEAD

HEADACHES/MIGRAINE

Headaches are usually caused by stress. Problems with the vertebrae in the neck arising from old whiplash injuries or poor posture are also frequently responsible. If headaches persist then medical advice should always be sought in case there is an underlying disorder. It may well be worth consulting an osteopath for spinal realignment.

Migraines are extremely painful, one-sided headaches usually accompanied by vomiting and an aversion to bright lights. Visual disturbances are also common. Sensitivity to certain foods such as cheese, chocolate and red wine; missed meals; tiredness and hormonal imbalances may also be contributory factors.

General advice
- Avoid stress and learn to relax
- Eat regularly
- Migraine sufferers should avoid substances suspected of inducing an attack
- Ensure that you have sufficient sleep

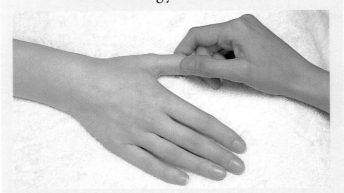

Reflexology Treatment

Head and brain

- Head and brain area
- Spine especially the neck
- Pituitary gland – to balance the hormones
- Solar plexus – to reduce stress
- Liver – to reduce nausea. The entire digestive system should be worked to encourage elimination
- Eyes

HEART PROBLEMS

ANGINA

Angina is caused by a lack of oxygen reaching the heart muscle due to coronary heart disease, high blood pressure or diseased heart valves. The symptoms are chest pain, which can radiate to the throat, upper jaw and left arm. Difficulty in breathing, sweating and dizziness may be experienced.

General advice
- Eat a healthy diet free from junk food, sugar, salt, fried foods and saturated animal fats. Increase your intake of fresh fruit, salads, vegetables, fibre and virgin olive oil
- Try to cut down on stress
- Take regular, gentle, physical exercise – e.g. Tai Chi, yoga or a 20 minute walk daily
- Give up smoking

Reflexology Treatment

- Heart area
- Lungs
- Diaphragm
- Solar plexus
- Adrenals

Heart

Lungs

Diaphragm

RESPIRATORY PROBLEMS

ASTHMA

The causes of asthma are varied and include allergies such as pollen, house dust, fur, feathers, certain foods or pollutants. Stress often precipitates an attack.

General advice
- Yoga is very beneficial as it encourages deeper breathing as well as reducing stress
- Avoid irritating substances

Reflexology Treatment

- Lung/chest area
- Solar plexus
- Diaphragm
- Adrenal glands – for allergies

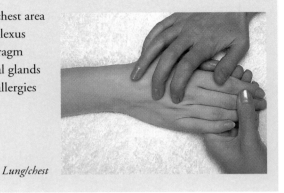

Lung/chest

COUGHS AND COLDS

Reflexology is not only an excellent way of relieving the symptoms of the common cold and speeding up recovery time but it is also remarkably effective at boosting the immune system. Regular reflexology greatly reduces the likelihood of catching a cold.

General advice
- Eat garlic, which is 'nature's antibiotic'
- Take at least one gram of vitamin C daily. Increase the dosage if you have a cold
- Eat ginger which helps to break down phlegm

Reflexology Treatment

- Lung/chest area – to break up the congestion and expel mucus
- Nose
- Throat
- Ears
- Eustacian tube
- Eyes
- Thymus – to boost the immune system
- Upper lymphatics

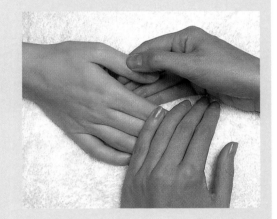

Nose

NASAL PROBLEMS

Nasal problems include acute or chronic catarrh, hay fever and sinusitis. Reflexology is renowned for its success with these problems. The most common causes are infections, allergies or the after effects of a cold.

General advice
- Avoid dairy foods, which encourage the production of mucus
- Steam inhalation with the addition of essential oils such as eucalyptus and cajeput

Reflexology Treatment

- Face area
- Sinuses
- Adrenals – to to counteract allergic responses
- Eyes and ears

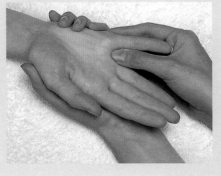

Sinuses

SKIN PROBLEMS

Skin problems include acne, eczema and psoriasis and the causes are debatable. Hormonal imbalances, stress and certain foods appear to play a major part.

General advice

* Eat a healthy diet with plenty of fresh fruit and vegetables
* Drink 6 – 8 glasses of water daily
* Avoid stress and learn to relax
* Avoid perfumed products. Use pure organic skin creams

Reflexology Treatment

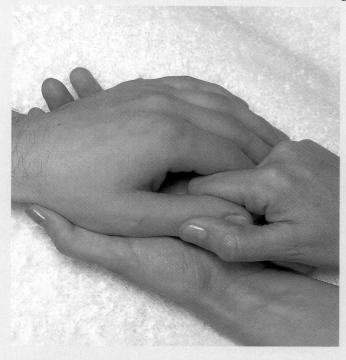

Face

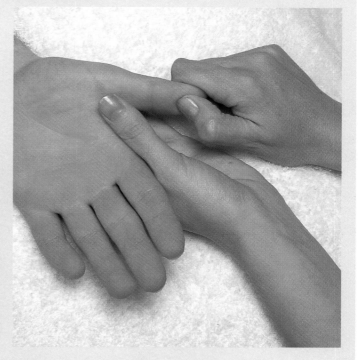

Pituitary Gland

* Reflex zones relating to the areas of the body affected e.g. face
* Pituitary gland – to balance the hormones
* Solar plexus – to relieve stress
* Adrenal glands – for stress and to counteract redness and itching
* Kidneys – to speed up elimination
* Lymphatics – to detoxify
* Digestive system – to encourage elimination

Conclusion

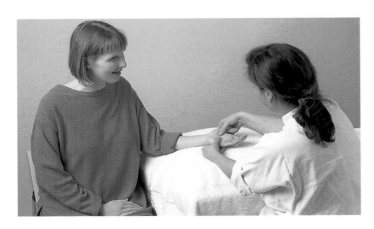

Both giving and receiving a reflexology treatment is a pleasurable experience.

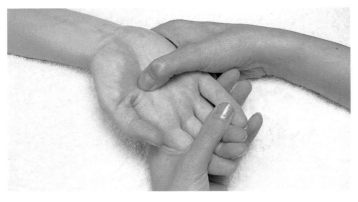

Reflexology is now regarded as an important complementary therapy.

This book has hopefully enabled you to carry out a complete hand reflexology treatment both on your friends and family as well as yourself. Without a doubt both giving and receiving a treatment can be immensely enjoyable and satisfying. Reflexology must surely be one of the most pleasurable therapies available and it has such marvellous effects on our health.

Perhaps you have been inspired to train as a professional reflexologist. Reflexology is rapidly expanding and fully qualified practitioners are very much in demand. Reflexology is no longer regarded as merely a 'New-Age' practice – rather it is now widely respected as an important complementary therapy, and plays a vital part in health care all over the world.

A recognised professional training course will take at least nine months and will involve a comprehensive study of anatomy and physiology as well as in-depth case studies. Make sure the course is accredited to a reputable association so that you do not waste money on a worthless piece of paper. Check out the principal to determine how experienced they are, and whether or not they still practice. It is only through clinical practice that knowledge is gained. Ask to visit the College and ask as many questions as you want. It should be possible for you to look at some of the student's work and even sit in on a class. Choose your course wisely as this is your future career.

Whether you take up reflexology professionally or use it purely for your family and friends, reflexology will certainly enrich your life for many years to come.

If you are unsure, it is always worth checking with the main reflexology institutes or organisations in your region or country.

PRIMARY REFLEXOLOGY ASSOCIATIONS

United Kingdom

Beaumont College of Natural Medicine
39-41 Hinton Road, Bournemouth, Dorset,
BH1 2EF, England
Tel: (44) 01202 708887

International Federation of Reflexologists
78 Edridge Road, Croydon, Surrey,
CR0 1EF, England
Tel: (44) 181 667 9458

United States

International Institute of Reflexology
PO Box 12642, St Petersburg, Florida, 33733-2642,
USA

Reflexology Association of America
4012 S Rainbow Boulevard, Box K585, Las Vegas,
Nevada 89103-2059, USA

CANADA

Reflexology Association of Canada (RAC)
Box 110, 541 Turnberry Street, Brussels, Ontario
N0G 1H0, Canada
Tel: (1) 519 887 9991   Fax: (1) 519 887 9792

AUSTRALIA

Reflexology Association of Australia
PO Box 366, Cammeray, NSW 2062, Australia
Tel: (61) 02 4721 4752

RIGHT HAND

RELAXATION TECHNIQUES

- Greeting the hand
- Stroking hand and lower arm
- Stroking hand – palm up/palm down
- Opening the hand
- Knuckling the palm
- Loosening the wrist
- Moving the wrist
- Wrist rolling
- Loosening the fingers and thumb
- Moving the fingers and thumb
- Solar plexus release
- Fingertip stroking

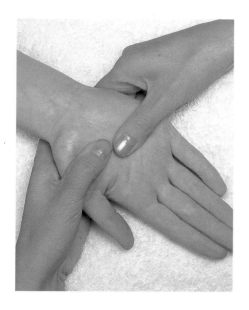

STEP BY STEP SEQUENCE

- Head and brain – thumb walk back and sides of thumb
- Pituitary gland – hook in and back – up on centre of thumb
- Face – thumb or finger walk front of thumb
- Neck – rotate base of thumb
- Neck/thyroid – thumb walk across back of base of thumb
- Neck/thyroid – finger walk across front of base of thumb
- Sinuses – walk down the back, sides and top of the fingers
- Teeth – walk down the front of the fingers
- Upper lymphatics – gently squeeze the webbing between each of the fingers
- Spine/sciatic line – caterpillar walk down the inside (thumb side) of the hand (spine) and above the wrist (sciatic line)
- Right eye and ear – thumb walk across ridge at base of fingers. Ear point (between fingers 4 and 5); eustachian tube (between fingers 3 and 4); eye point (between index and middle finger).
- Right lung – thumb walk upper third of palm of hand (to diaphragm line).
- Right lung/breast/mammary glands – finger walk down front of hand from base of fingers to diaphragm line

- Liver/gallbladder – thumb walk zones 5 - 3 between diaphragm line and waistline.
  Hook in and back-up technique on gallbladder reflex.
- Stomach/pancreas/duodenum – thumb walk zones 1 - 3 between diaphragm line and waistline
- Right adrenal gland – hook in and back-up
- Right kidney/ureter tube/bladder – pressure circles over kidney point, turn thumb and walk down towards inside of hand to bladder.
- Small intestines – thumb walk zones 1 - 4
- Ileocaecal valve/ascending/transverse colon – hook in and back-up on ileocaecal valve, walk up the ascending colon and across transverse colon
- Joints – right shoulder/elbow/hip/knee/ – thumb walk down outer edge of hand
- Right ovary – rotate on reflex point on outside of the wrist
- Uterus/prostate – rotate on reflex point on inside of wrist
- Right fallopian tube/vas deferens/lymph nodes of groin – thumb walk across back and front of wrist
- Stroke right hand

LEFT HAND

RELAXATION TECHNIQUES

- Greeting the hand
- Stroking hand and lower arm
- Stroking hand – palm up/palm down
- Opening the hand
- Knuckling the palm
- Loosening the wrist
- Moving the wrist
- Wrist rolling
- Loosening the fingers and thumb
- Moving the fingers and thumb
- Fingertip stroking
- Solar plexus release

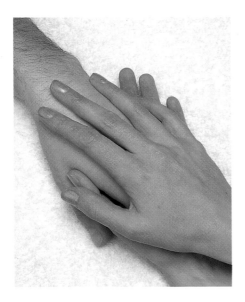

CLOSING MOVEMENTS

STEP BY STEP SEQUENCE

- Head and brain – thumb walk back and sides of thumb
- Pituitary gland – hook in and back-up on centre of thumb
- Face – thumb/finger walk front of thumb
- Neck – rotate base of thumb
- Neck/thyroid – thumb walk across back of base of thumb
- Neck/thyroid – Walk across front of base of thumb
- Sinuses – walk down the back, sides and top of the fingers
- Teeth – walk down the front of the fingers
- Upper lymphatics – gently squeeze the webbing between each of the fingers
- Spine/sciatic line – caterpillar walk down the inside (thumb side) of the hand (spine) and above the wrist (sciatic line)
- Right eye and ear – thumb walk across ridge at base of fingers. Eye point (between index and middle finger), eustachian tube (between fingers 3 and 4), ear point (between fingers 4 and 5)
- Left lung – thumb walk upper third of palm of hand (to diaphragm line)
- Left lung/breast/mammary glands – finger walk down front of upper third of hand from base of fingers to diaphragm line

- Heart area – pressure circles on cardiac area and circular massage
- Stomach/pancreas/duodenum – thumb walk zones 1 - 3 between diaphragm line and waistline
- Spleen – thumb walk zones 5 - 4
- Left adrenal gland – hook in and back-up
- Left kidney/ureter tube/bladder – pressure circles over kidney point, turn thumb and work down towards inside of hand to bladder
- Small intestines – thumb walk zones 1 - 4
- Transverse/descending/sigmoid colon/rectum – walk across waistline zones 1 - 5, change hands to walk down descending colon, turn thumb 90° to walk across sigmoid colon and in to the rectum.
- Joints – left shoulder/elbow/hip/ankle – thumb walk down outer edge of hand
- Left ovary – rotate on reflex point on outside of wrist
- Uterus/prostate – rotate on reflex point on inside of wrist
- Left fallopian tube/vas deferens/lymph nodes of groin – thumb walk across back and front of wrist
- Stroke left hand

- Return to any areas which were sensitive
- Perform any of your favourite relaxation techniques – use oil/cream if desired
- Run fingertips lightly over both hands
- Clasp both hands gently
- Cover up hands and allow the receiver to relax
- Offer a glass of water for and encourage receiver to drink 6 - 8 glasses over the next 24 hour

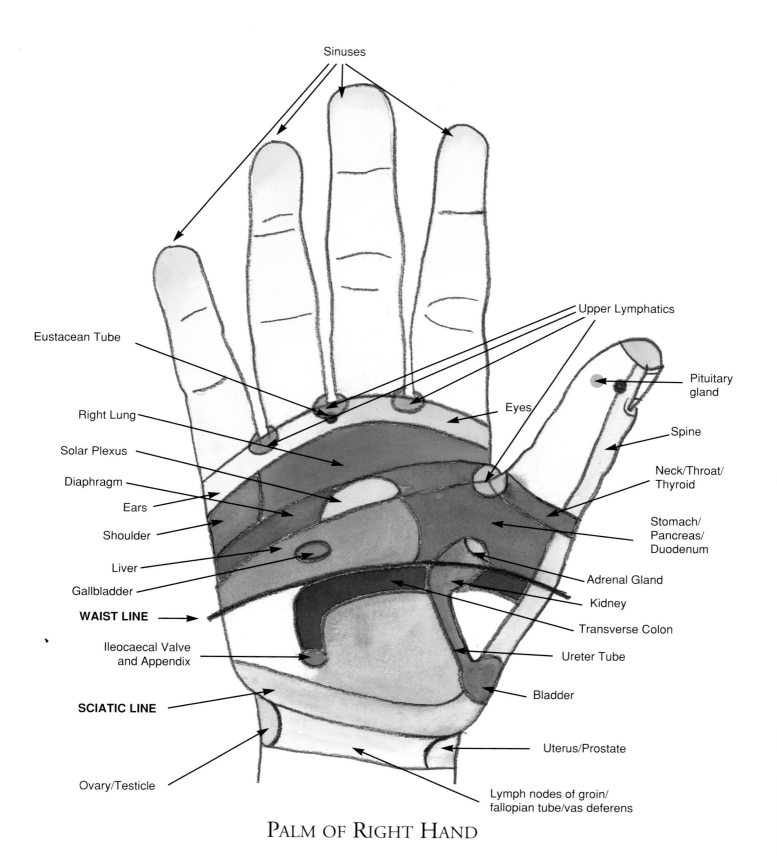

Sinuses

Upper Lymphatics

Eustacean Tube

Pituitary gland

Eyes

Right Lung

Spine

Solar Plexus

Neck/Throat/ Thyroid

Diaphragm

Ears

Stomach/ Pancreas/ Duodenum

Shoulder

Liver

Adrenal Gland

Gallbladder

Kidney

WAIST LINE

Transverse Colon

Ileocaecal Valve and Appendix

Ureter Tube

SCIATIC LINE

Bladder

Uterus/Prostate

Ovary/Testicle

Lymph nodes of groin/ fallopian tube/vas deferens

PALM OF RIGHT HAND

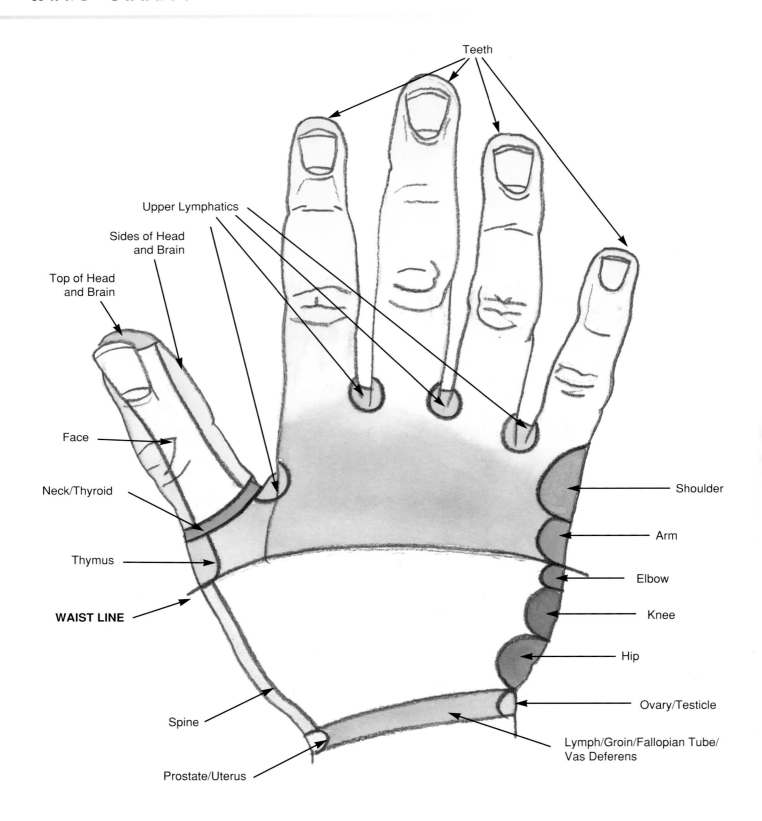

Teeth

Upper Lymphatics

Sides of Head
and Brain

Top of Head
and Brain

Face

Neck/Thyroid

Thymus

WAIST LINE

Spine

Prostate/Uterus

Shoulder

Arm

Elbow

Knee

Hip

Ovary/Testicle

Lymph/Groin/Fallopian Tube/
Vas Deferens

BACK OF THE RIGHT HAND

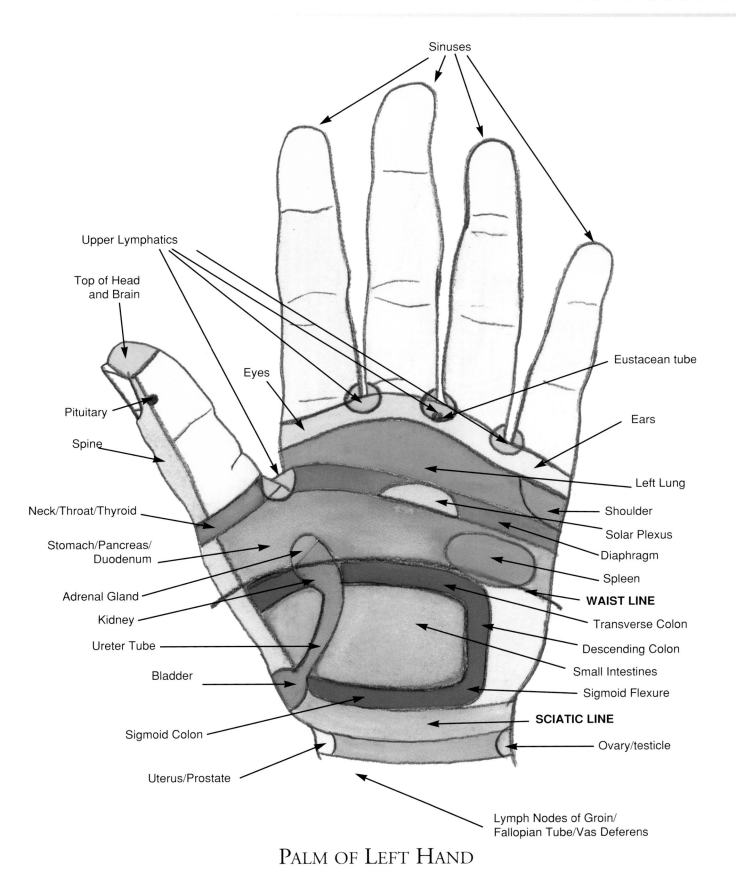

Sinuses

Upper Lymphatics

Top of Head
and Brain

Eyes

Eustacean tube

Pituitary

Ears

Spine

Left Lung

Neck/Throat/Thyroid

Shoulder

Solar Plexus

Stomach/Pancreas/
Duodenum

Diaphragm

Spleen

Adrenal Gland

WAIST LINE

Kidney

Transverse Colon

Ureter Tube

Descending Colon

Small Intestines

Bladder

Sigmoid Flexure

SCIATIC LINE

Sigmoid Colon

Ovary/testicle

Uterus/Prostate

Lymph Nodes of Groin/
Fallopian Tube/Vas Deferens

PALM OF LEFT HAND

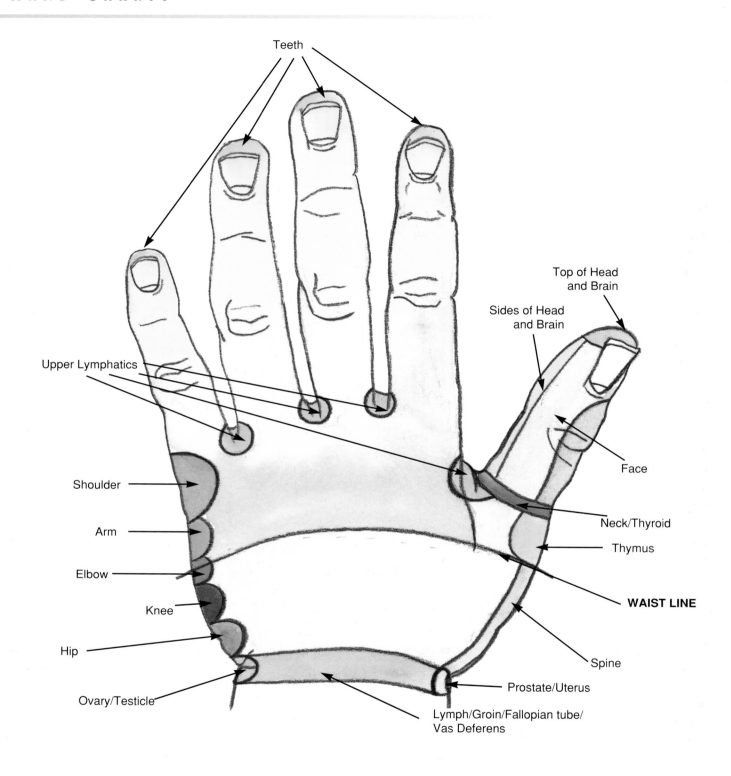

Teeth

Top of Head
and Brain

Sides of Head
and Brain

Upper Lymphatics

Face

Shoulder

Neck/Thyroid

Arm

Thymus

Elbow

WAIST LINE

Knee

Hip

Spine

Ovary/Testicle

Prostate/Uterus

Lymph/Groin/Fallopian tube/
Vas Deferens

BACK OF THE LEFT HAND

Index

All Pictures © Quantum Books Ltd.

Many thanks to the models:
Adam, Maria and Sarah.